D0494719

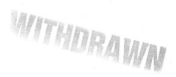

Managing in Health Care

Pearson
Education

We work with leading authors to develop the
strongest educational materials on social science,
bringing cutting-edge thinking and best
learning practice to a global market.

Under a range of well-known imprints, including
Prentice Hall, we craft high quality and
electronic publications which help readers to understand
and apply their content, whether studying or at work.

To find out more about the complete range of our
publishing, please visit us on the World Wide Web at:
www.pearsoneduc.com

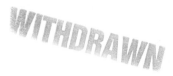

Managing in Health Care

A Guide for Nurses, Midwives and Health Visitors

Lesley Dowding (Principal Lecturer in Nursing Studies, Coventry University)
and
Jill Barr (Principal Lecturer in Nursing and Midwifery, De Montfort University)

Prentice
Hall

An imprint of **Pearson Education**

London · New York · San Francisco · Toronto · Sydney
Tokyo · Singapore · Hong Kong · Cape Town · Madrid
Paris · Milan · Munich · Amsterdam

Pearson Education Limited
Edinburgh Gate
Harlow
Essex CM20 2JE

and Associated Companies throughout the world

Visit us on the World Wide Web at:
www.pearsoneduc.com

First published 2002

ISBN 0582 38235 1

British Library Cataloguing-in-Publication Data
A catalogue record for this book is available from the British Library

10 9 8 7 6 5 4 3 2 1
05 04 03 02

Typeset in 10/12.5pt Sabon by 30
Printed and bound in Malaysia ·

Contents

Preface

There can be little doubt that the reforms of the last few decades within the National Health Service have had a major impact on the management responsibilities in nursing, midwifery and health visiting. The theory of management itself may be seen as someone else's business because the term 'management' is perceived in the context of a group of people in a hierarchy rather than as a higher order skill. The purpose of this book is to provide student nurses with a textbook that demonstrates how the concepts and principles of management are intrinsically linked to the work that nurses do. This book will therefore be of relevance to all students in pre-registration programmes and those meeting management theory for the first time.

The text will unpack the role of nurses, midwives and health visitors and illustrate the links with management principles. It will start by examining student experiences in caring and progress through to the development of the individual working within the health care organisation.

Wherever registered professionals work there will be a management structure and it is important that nurses, midwives and health visitors have the opportunity to develop the skills necessary to make management decisions appropriate to the needs of the client group and the context of health care where they practise.

An incremental and systematic approach is taken in the development of the knowledge and practice of management skills. The book will examine three main areas related to student and qualified nurses, midwives and health visitors in terms of them as an individual, working in a team, and in the business of health care.

This is intended to help students and practitioners to recognise the need to manage in complex health care settings, in a society that is becoming more consumer and business orientated and where health care expectations are rising at an incredible pace.

This book is designed to be used either as a main text or as a distance learning tool in that it contains useful exercises to enable the student to understand a variety of aspects of management theory and their application within the clinical area. Similarly, it aims to help students of nursing, midwifery and health visiting grasp management principles in the context of their everyday professional lives. The book is recommended for use in conjunction with 'purist' management texts and seeks to aid the application of those theories to professional practice.

Acknowledgements

There are several people we would wish to thank for their help, support and contributions during the production of this work: family and friends – Bunny and Hilary Dowding, Jim Barr, Rav and Sue Jayram; special thanks to Sue White for the cartoons/graphics to show us and the readers a different perspective on applying management theory to professional practice, and local critical readers Kevin Cole and Alistair Hewison. Without their help this book would not have been possible.

Publisher's Acknowledgements

We are grateful to the following for permission to reproduce copyright material:

Figure 2.2 from *Techniques of Structured Problem Solving, 2nd Edition*, published by Van Nostrand Reinhold, reprinted by permission of the author (VanGundy, A. B. 1988); Figure 2.3 from *Culture's Consequences: International Differences in Work Related Values*, published by Sage, Inc., copyright Geert Hofstede, reproduced with permission of the author (Hofstede, G. 1980); Table 5.4 from *The Named Nurse in Practice*, copyright 1997, reprinted by permission of the WB Saunders (Dargan, R. 1997); Figure 53.6 from *The Multi-Disciplinary Team*, reproduced by kind permission of the King's Fund, London (McFarlane, J. K. 1980); Figure 6.1 after Figure in *Action Centered Leadership*, published by Gower Publishing Ltd, reprinted by permission of the author (Adair, J. 1979); Table 6.1 from *Leadership Roles and Management Functions in Nursing: Theory and Application, 2nd Edition*, reprinted by permission of Lippincott Williams and Wilkins (Marquis, B. L. and Huston, C. J. 1996); Table 7.1 from *Organisational Behaviour: Concepts and Applications, 3rd Edition*, copyright 1984, reprinted by permission of Pearson Education, Inc., Upper Saddle River, NJ (Gray, J. L. and Starke, F. A. 1984); Figure 7.2 from *Management and Organisational Behaviour, 5th Edition* reprinted by permission of Pearson Education Ltd (Mullins, L. J. 1999); Table 8.2 from *On Death and Dying*, published by Tavistock Publications, reprinted by permission of Taylor & Francis Books Ltd (Kubler Ross, E. 1970);

Table 10.1 from *From Cradle to Grave: Fifty Years of the NHS*, reproduced by kind permission of the King's Fund, London (Rivett, G. 1998); Table 12.4 from *Fitness for Practice*, reprinted by permission of the United Kingdom Central Council for Nursing, Midwifery and Health Visiting (UKCC 1999); Figure 12.6 from *Making a Difference: Strengthening the Nursing, Midwifery and Health Visitor Contribution to Health and Healthcare* (HMSO 1999), Crown copyright material is reproduced under Class Licence Number C01W0000039 with the permission of the Controller of HMSO and ther Queeen's Printer for Scotland.

While every effort has been made to trace the owners of copyright material, in a few cases this has proved impossible and we take this opportunity to offer our apologies to any copyright holders whose rights we have unwittingly infringed.

Part

I

The individual

1

Getting Started

By the end of this chapter you will have had the opportunity to:

- recognise the importance of self-awareness within a health care environment
- undertake a SWOT analysis in order to develop a meaningful career path
- discuss the advantages and disadvantages of various time management strategies
- describe the difficulties of coping with stress and the systems that may contribute to its successful management.

Introduction

Whenever patients and clients comment about the quality of care they receive from health care professionals they are referring to how that care has been organised and delivered, by whom and to what standard. This suggests that there is a connection between the ability of the nurses, midwives and health visitors to manage and the quality of care that is being delivered in a particular environment. In order to manage care effectively and efficiently it is important for those involved in the delivery of that care first to acquire an awareness of themselves as people and, second to have personal goals, aims and objectives to work towards.

This chapter aims to provide the building blocks for nurses, midwives and health visitors to develop a career route or pathway. It will address issues of self-awareness; the identification of individual strengths and weaknesses; goal setting; time management; coping with stress; and managing support systems.

Self-awareness

There is no single definition of self-awareness but it may be seen as a dynamic state of mind that a person reaches after examining their strengths and weaknesses in individual abilities, attributes, and roles. It involves the influences and reactions from significant others and may be dependent on time and place. Within a caring profession it is important that we are aware of the image we portray to our patients, as it is one of the major factors that encourages or detracts from the healing process. Sometimes assumptions about ourselves do not correspond with the perceptions of others, but when considering our own views and those of others the overall effect is to help us to develop self-awareness. York (1995) indicated that self-awareness should imply that the individual:

- has reached a balanced and as honest a view as possible of his/her abilities and limitations without overestimating or underestimating self;
- is aware that his/her behaviour always has effects on others and may, therefore, regularly need modification to achieve effective communication and relationships;
- takes positive steps to ascertain the views of others about his/her behaviours and takes particular note of any consensus of views. (York 1995)

There are numerous issues where self-awareness and self-knowledge will be of help to nurses, midwives and health visitors: attitudes and beliefs about abortion; single parents; euthanasia; and refusal of treatment, to name but a few. However, irrespective of a nurse's own beliefs and values, a nurse may not refuse to care for a patient except in certain circumstances, e.g. a nurse may refuse to help with the actual abortion, but following this the patient's needs override any personal view that the nurse may hold.

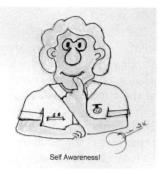

Self Awareness!

It may be useful to identify stressful elements within your daily life and you should be encouraged to develop networks, which may include partners, friends, colleagues or relatives, to assist in reducing the effects of stressors. Awareness of one's capabilities and limitations is particularly important when considering a career where interaction with the general public at a time of illness, stress or trauma is a feature. Most of life involves interpersonal relationships of one sort or another, so there is a clear need for effective communication and collaboration if one is to take responsibility in attaining the goals of life.

In interpersonal terms, self-awareness concerns perceptions that have been highlighted within a model known as Johari's Window (see Figure 1.1). This describes the perceptual differences and possible conflicts of behaviour that were identified by two psychologists, Joe Luft and Harry Ingham (York 1995). The window has four 'panes' which relate to aspects of self. It can be said that by identifying the areas or traits of oneself related to areas 1–3, then the elements that make up area 4 will inevitably become smaller. This makes individuals more able in terms of ability to consider the effects of their behaviour on others and the identification of positive steps that might be

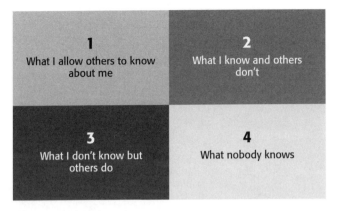

Figure 1.1 Johari's Window
Adapted from York (1995)

taken in order to effect an improvement. So self-awareness can be used as a significant force for developing and improving individuals, helping them make sound decisions for life and working careers and developing important skills in interpersonal relationships.

While self-awareness is important for personal and interpersonal purposes, it is vital when work involves any form of leadership. If one is to become an effective leader then it can only be achieved by knowing oneself and the impact one has on others (Chapter 7). The only people who can give managers reliable feedback about leadership style and the effect that it has on the workforce are the members of that workforce. However, this can be extremely difficult, particularly if the workforce does not see the leader in a favourable light and if that leader has the power to 'hire and fire'. Wherever possible an exercise of self-analysis, should be carried out. The leader could describe themselves in terms of their main characteristics; following this they could ask the views of 'safe' but honest people or relatives to do the same thing. Then, by comparing the views, an overall picture will be developed. It must be recognised that traits demonstrated at work may not necessarily be demonstrated at home. Similarly the converse may be true. This is an excellent method of gaining insight into self and using it as a tool for improvement.

Strengths and weaknesses

Occasionally it is useful to take a long, hard look at yourself and what better time than at the start of your career in health care. It is relatively easy to identify your perceived weaknesses, but when it comes to strengths things are a little more difficult. It is only by identifying these two elements that you can go on to consider your opportunities for yourself and identify the threats that may stop you from achieving your overall goal. Figure 1.2 shows the elements of a SWOT analysis and the format it may take.

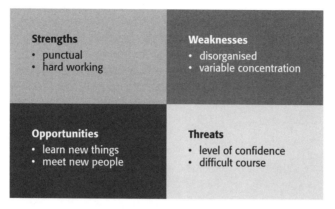

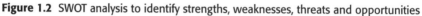

Strengths	Weaknesses
• punctual • hard working	• disorganised • variable concentration
Opportunities • learn new things • meet new people	**Threats** • level of confidence • difficult course

Figure 1.2 SWOT analysis to identify strengths, weaknesses, threats and opportunities

- Take a few moments to look at yourself in order to undertake a SWOT analysis.
- Keep your findings in the personal part of your portfolio to examine occasionally and see if you are still on the right track.

This type of analysis helps to indicate where you might have strengths to develop and where you might have a weakness, so you will always be on the lookout for opportunities. Clearly if you have done this sort of exercise you will be able to demonstrate your talents more easily in order to get results. It is also most impressive when this exercise forms part of your application for jobs in the future.

Objectives and goals

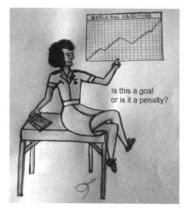

As part of getting yourself organised it is important to decide what you want to do and achieve at work. This approach is similar to the way you engage with your patients and clients as part of care and therapeutic interventions. It is important, however, to think carefully about personal, professional and academic pursuits and interests on the basis of a time scale that is realistic and therefore achievable. This time scale may be viewed from either a long-term or a short-term perspective.

How would you define the following in terms of time?

1 long-term goals
2 medium-term goals
3 short-term goals.

For some of you your long-term goal might be as long as twenty years away, but for others it may be just the three years that it takes to get through training and become a registered nurse. From a practical point of view, planning for goals and objectives may involve other colleagues, a mentor or a supervisor, e.g. helping with reflective practice. This process of identifying, analysing and deciding what you want to accomplish for yourself will help you to focus your ideas and consequently your time and effort in getting organised. From a professional angle, factors for consideration in planning your goals and objectives are the job description and the business plan of your unit or organisation that you are working for or seeking employment with. Other factors that may be considered are your appraisal by your immediate line manager and the development of your personal portfolio. Adair (1987) suggests that a sense of purpose and a sense of direction can be developed although they can be modified in the light of experience so it can be seen that objectives are not '*set in tablets of stone*' but may be adapted according to your environmental changes.

Time management

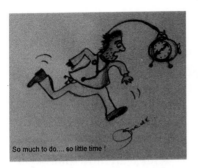

So much to do.... so little time !

According to Adair (1990), all planning is about thinking forward in time. However, plans vary both in terms of time scale and in their precision. In relation to getting yourself organised, the effective management of your time can contribute to the development of managerial skills. This is dependent on whether you are able to complete your work on time and to the standard that is expected from you according to your experience and role expectations/stages of training.

List five activities that you do in order to use your time effectively.

There are a variety of ideas and factors that you can consider in order to make sure that you are making the best use of your time at work and elsewhere. These include making a daily list of things that you have to do; assessing the order of priority for the tasks; using of a diary or timetable (Figure 1.3) both for planning and as a log book; and the allocation of time for specific and particular jobs to which you are committed to.

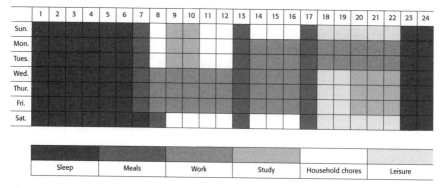

Figure 1.3 Example of timetable for effective time management

Information technology can provide additional support for you to manage your time more effectively both in terms of managing information and in decision making. Remember that 'we all find time to do what we really want to do' (Adair 1990).

Stress and coping

Stress is part of everyday life; whether it be at home or in the workplace, we must take measures to cope with it. Selye (1976) says that stress is 'essentially reflected by the rate of all wear and tear caused by life'. But what is stress? It is very difficult to define as it may mean different things to different people. Whatever your own definition, it is probably expressed as something negative which will have an adverse effect on you as a person. Selye (1976) talks about good and bad stress (eustress and distress). He says that we need a certain amount of eustress in order to lead an active, healthy life. It is the point at which the increasing levels of stress become harmful that requires recognition.

> Take a few moments to jot down a list of sources of stress in your life.

In all probability the majority of these relate to work and/or study. Many studies have been undertaken that relate to the causes of stress including Melia (1987), Lindop (1991) and Lees and Ellis (1990). You might like to examine any of these to gain further insight.

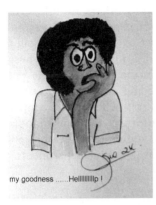

my goodness ......Hellllllllp !

Don't forget all the stressful things that occur outside work, e.g. the children fighting over the computer, the toast burning at breakfast time, etc. Holmes and Rahe (1967) produced a well-known table of events that showed that increased amounts of stress had the knock-on effect of increasing absenteeism or sickness. Irrespective of the cause of stress, Oakley (1992) found that birth complications were fewer in women who had high levels of social support. Similarly, Antoni et al (1998) suggest that offering psychological interventions that provide support and teach coping strategies may be beneficial. We only have to look at the upsurge of associations to see the value of these in times of stress, e.g. the Stillbirth & Neonatal Death Society (SANDS), the Miscarriage Association, the Diabetic Association, etc; the list covers a wide variety of illnesses/conditions/ situations.

Accepting that stress is a part of our lives and that it is unlikely to go away, it is important that we recognise signs in ourselves as well as in others, and that we develop coping strategies. Stress can manifest itself in a variety of ways, many of which are behavioural in nature, e.g. early morning waking, restlessness and irritability, and physiologically as insomnia, palpitations, raised cardiac output, raised blood pressure, raised metabolic rate and hyperventilation. Lazarus and Folkman (1984) talk of two different strategies, which they have called:

- problem-focused coping
- emotion-focused coping.

Problem-focused coping involves a conscious action, e.g. collecting as much information as possible about the stressor in order to reduce fear of the unknown; developing a new skill, e.g. attending a time management course to manage work and home life effectively.

Emotion-focused coping, on the other hand, involves an unconscious action. Lazarus (1999) suggests a number of defence mechanisms including denial, identification, displacement, repression, reaction formulation, projection and intellectualisation. In reality people probably use both types of coping strategies and it is part of the role of the professional to recognise them and help people to cope effectively with their stress.

Support systems

There are a variety of support systems that are available to aid and support newly qualified practitioners. Some are formal while others are informal. Formal support systems include mentors and clinical supervisors, and access to them will be organised by the line manager and according to the policy and procedure that will be in place in the organisational context. These formal mechanisms are effective to support you in the pursuit of aims and objectives, which are directly related to your role and post. Of course you will still be able to access any member of trained staff when in the clinical area if your allocated mentor is not available. Informal help and support could be obtained from friends and colleagues. In addition some employers offer the facility of independent counsellors via their personnel departments.

Conclusion

Throughout this chapter you have been asked to identify how you see yourself and are seen by others. This is often a difficult task because we do not usually like to identify our strengths. It is important to recognise how you present yourself and how you have changed or will change as you go through the course of study. Nursing, in whatever arena, is largely about communication and instilling faith in people who are at their most vulnerable. It is also a time when you may be feeling pressured to comply or perform duties previously unknown to you.

Summary of key points

This chapter has briefly looked at various aspects of self-awareness in order that you are able to progress through the course to become the best registered nurse, midwife or health visitor that you can.

- **Self-awareness:** Focused on what this is and how you might become more aware of the image you portray in order to deliver quality care to your patients/clients. Furthermore we examined Johari's Window in order to consider the effect your behaviour might have on others.

- **Strengths and weaknesses:** Went on to look at ways in which you can identify your own strengths and weaknesses via a SWOT analysis. This exercise is of tremendous use when applying for jobs in the future as you will be asked to write about yourself through supporting information.

- **Objectives and goals:** Again it is important to set ourselves short-, medium-, and long-term goals. The short-term goals help you to attain a sense of achievement whereas the longer-term ones give you a more enduring sense of purpose.

- **Time management:** Planning successfully is vital if you are to attain your goals. We all have times when we put everything off until the last minute but by using an effective plan you can reduce the stress of having to produce work by a specific time.

- **Stress and coping:** Here we looked at the effects of stress, recognising that we need a little stress in order to function effectively.

- **Support systems:** Are vital if you are to survive. This section gave you some idea of the who and the how to develop these systems in order to ensure that you cope well with the course.

References

Adair J (1990) *Great Leaders*, Talbot Adair Press

Antoni M H, Schneiderman N. Ironson G (1998) Stress, Management for HIV-infection in Johnson H C, Hayes A M, Field T M, Schneiderman N, McCabe P M (2000) *Stress, Coping and Emotion*, Lawrence Erlbaum Associates

Holmes D S, Rahe R H (1967) The social readjustment rating scale, *Journal of Psychometric Research*, 11:213 –18, 469

Lazarus R (1999) *Stress and Emotion*, Free Association Press

Lazarus R S, Folkman S (1984) *Stress and Coping*, Springer.

Lees S, Ellis N (1990) The design of a stress-management programme for Nursing Personnel, *Journal of Advanced Nursing*, no. 8, vol. 15, p. 964

Lindop E (1991) Individual stress amongst nurses in training: why some leave while others stay, *Nurse Education Today*, no. 2, vol. 11, pp. 110–120

Melia K (1987) Balance of Power, *Nursing Times*, no. 25, vol. 83, pp. 36–39

Oakley A (1992) *Social Support and Motherhood: the natural history of a research project*, Blackwell Publishers

Selye H (1976) *The Stress of Life* (2nd edn) McGraw-Hill

York A (1995) *Managing for Success: A Human Approach*, Cassell in association with the ISM

Further reading

Armstrong M (1990) *Management Processes and Functions*, Institute of Personnel Management

Faulkner A (1985) *Nursing – A Creative Approach*, Baillière Tindall

Gross R D (1987) *Psychology: The Science of Mind and Behaviour*, Hodder & Stoughton

Iles V (1997) *Really Managing Health Care*, Open University Press

Makin P, Cooper C, Cox C (1989) *Managing People at Work*, The British Psychological Society and Routledge

McGhie A (1986) *Psychology as Applied to Nursing* (8th edn) Churchill Livingstone

McKenna E (1994) *Business Psychology & Organisational Behaviour: A Students' Handbook*, Lawrence Erlbaum Associates

Millar B, Burnard P (1994) *Critical Care Nursing*, Ballière Tindall

Palmer A, Burns S, Bulman C (1994) *Reflective Practice in Nursing*, Blackwell Science

Quinn F M (1995) *The Principles and Practice of Nurse Education* (3rd edn) Chapman & Hall

Schön D A (1987) *The Reflective Practitioner: How Professionals Think in Action*, Basic Books Inc.

Sperling A (1957) *Psychology Made Simple*, W H Allen

Sullivan E J, Decker P J (1997) *Effective Leadership and Management in Nursing* (4th edn) Addison-Wesley

Weber A L (1992) *Social Psychology*, Harper Perennial

Williams H (1994) *The Essence of Managing People*, Prentice Hall

2

Decision making

By the end of this chapter you will have had the opportunity to:

- identify the importance of problem solving and decision making in health care
- discuss the value of some of the problem-solving models in health care
- utilise some problem-solving and decision-making methods in order to enhance your health care management.

Introduction

Nurses, midwives and health visitors are involved with problems on an hourly basis as part of their work. Their patients and clients may have health issues or problems and the people with whom they work may have personal and professional problems. Health care organisations also rely on and demand from their staff a capacity to deal with issues and make decisions. Staff may, however, be faced with constraints such as time and money for effective organisation and delivery of health care. Stewart's (1989, 1996) model of a job can be useful in seeing how nurses, midwives and health visitors view the constraints they face in their daily work (see Figure 2.1). It can be seen that as the demands get larger and more constraints are imposed, then choices for problem solving diminish. It is therefore important that we learn how to deal with the world of problems, decision making and problem solving. Indeed, Benner (1984) highlighted that decision making was the main criterion for judging expert professional nursing practice.

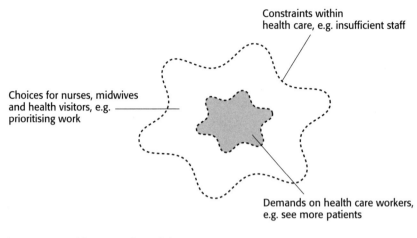

Figure 2.1 Healthcare work model
Adapted from Stewart (1989)

Concepts of problem solving and decision making

Problem solving and decision making are not seen as the same concept, although it may be inferred that they are the same. Problem solving is a broader concept than just decision making. This chapter will focus on two main areas:

1. The concept of problems in health care.
2. The concept of decision making in health care.

Definitions of the concept of 'problem' focus on ideas such as a mismatch or difficulty in choosing between different alternatives. 'A problem can be defined as any situation in which a gap is perceived to exist between what is and what should be' (VanGundy 1988 p. 3).

The idea that 'problems only really arise when an experience is troubling an individual' is central to the idea of problem solving. As a student you will recognise that problems are not confined to health care, and you will have had and will have your own share of personal problems and decisions to make.

> Identify some of the problems you faced when you were looking for a course to study.

Some of those problems may have been related to whether you could cope with the extra academic work or may have been related to finances. How were you going to live on a bursary or a grant? The cost of the course, travelling and books needed may also have added to your worries. Another

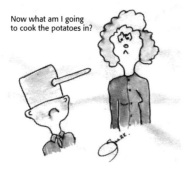

Now what am I going to cook the potatoes in?

problem may have been related to the need for supportive relationships. When you have a home to run, children to organise or the responsibilities of caring for and supporting family members you do need to identify your own practical and emotional needs when embarking on a course. Problem solving involves identifying the type of problem, looking at how it may affect you, the choices you face and the consequences of the decisions you make. Decision making is therefore the part of problem solving that is concerned with the choice of solutions and/or actions where a difficulty *or* an opportunity arise.

Types of problems

Interestingly, Armstrong (1990) identified that there are no real problems, only opportunities. This is an optimistic way of looking at managing life and gives us a positive approach to our professional and personal life. Student days in nursing are not going to be easy. There will be times when you will want to blame and criticise others in order that you can cope with the day-to-day hurdles. You may have heard the saying 'no pain, no gain' and it has to be said that in health care, the difficulties in the unravelling of problems for ourselves and our patients/clients and even looking ahead to *find* problems will ultimately bring satisfaction for you when you know that your patients value your work.

VanGundy (1988) suggested that problem-solving success depended on two factors:

1. the nature of the problem, *and*
2. the approaches used.

There will be problems that may be regarded as trivial or simple and then there will be more complex and serious problems. The less complex problems can be dealt with in a more routine fashion or use of a 'rule of thumb' approach. For instance, if you forget money for lunch, you may have four options:

1. Ask a colleague for a loan.
2. Go home for lunch.
3. Go to the cash point.
4. Go hungry!

These types of problems have *certainty* about what the issues are and what the outcomes are likely to be. Other problems are less certain. There is an element of the unknown about them and often you do not have full information necessary to solve them. Sometimes you can use logical methods to solve them but sometimes they are even more complex and you may have to use creative problem-solving methods. This reflects two broad approaches in management:

1. The rational (scientific) approach.
2. The creative (intuitive) approach.

Hamm (1988) felt that, rather than considering these two as separate methods, they could be seen as both ends of a continuum with decision making occurring somewhere along that continuum. It was also felt that the more time and information that were available, the nearer to the rational end of the continuum the decision making would be.

Try to list some examples of clinical problems in your area where decisions are needed from both management approaches.

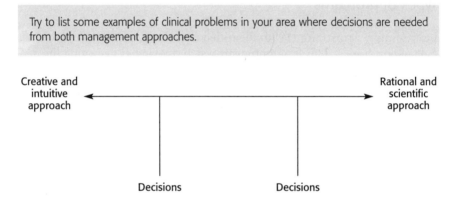

Figure 2.2 Approaches to problem solving and decision making

You may have thought that those problems that are long term, human and complex may be better solved using both rational and creative approaches. One example may be helping a family with a child with learning disabilities to look at choices of schooling. They may need to come to a decision, knowing the constraints of local authority resources, travelling concerns and social acceptability issues. It may be about helping a new mother to breastfeed twins and manage going back to work after three months. These problems require decisions based on individual needs and creative solutions will sometimes be required.

We will now look at another example which is a pertinent problem in all disciplines in health care.

Sister Jenkins is in charge of Elfin Ward. She receives four telephone calls one evening when staff call in to report sickness and an inability to do their shifts the next day. She notes that this is happening a little too regularly.

She needs to make *decisions* on how to cover the ward the next day. She asks staff on duty if they want extra shifts. Two part-time staff reluctantly agree to work. She then *decides* to contact bank staff. There are no available staff who agree to work. She then *decides* to telephone the agency and eventually two staff are found to cover.

Sister Jenkins has made some management decisions.

Now think about the problem as a whole and write some notes about Sister Jenkins' problems.

You may have thought about whether this was really as simple a problem as getting more staff to cover the shift or you may have wondered whether there was an epidemic of influenza in the area and this problem was beyond Sister Jenkins' control. You may have wondered at the difference between problem solving and decision making. Problem solving really looks at the 'big picture' of the issues and the decisions that have to be made. Problem identification as a stage involves *separating the problem from its symptoms*. Peter Drucker (1964) highlights the fact that this is often forgotten: 'the most common source of mistakes in management decisions is the emphasis on finding the right answer rather than the right question'. Searching for the right question means asking systematic questions about the perceived problem.

Remember then that the *problem itself* needs to be analysed and separated from the *symptoms*. It is important, however, to look at who should be involved with the problem analysis.

Problem solvers and problem owners

Health care professionals will solve problems in many different contexts. Sometimes they will need to think of solutions in an emergency setting where time is of the essence, for instance in the case of severe haemorrhage or other life-threatening situations. At other times, there may be time to work through health care goals and therapies with patients and clients in a less rushed atmosphere. In other cases there may be a need to work through the problems with a variety of other professionals and the quality of the solutions

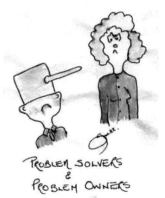

PROBLEM SOLVERS
&
PROBLEM OWNERS

may arise out of a period of reflection and collaboration with others. It is useful therefore to identify who might *own* or be affected by the problem, or even be affected by any solution. This group would be known as the problem owners.

There may be a need to use a variety of skills to solve problems from logical thinking, intuition or trial and error, depending on the problem or the context of the specific problem. The kind of management skills and styles you have may affect the outcome of the solution and decisions made. Vroom and Yetton (1973) identified different styles of problem solvers depending on their position on a management style continuum (see Decision-making methods box below). Their style of problem solving depended on who they involved in the problem-solving process and how they involved them.

Decision-making methods (examples of types)

A1 Solve problems and make decisions yourselves using available information
A11 Get information from subordinates and solve problem yourself
C1 Share problem with individual subordinates, generate solutions, then make your own decision
C11 Share problem with subordinate groups, generate suggestions then make your own decisions
G11 Share the problem with subordinate groups, generate ideas and come to a consensus on a solution

(Vroom and Yetton 1973)

A leader of any group is dependent on the ability to 'fit' with the people in that particular organisation and the type of work undertaken. A successful leader in one clinical area will not necessarily be a success in another area. Organisational culture in the particular health service areas will affect the leadership success. The culture of an operating theatre is very different to that of a rehabilitation ward and also to the culture of community midwifery. Organisational culture in this instance refers to the shared values, attitudes and beliefs of the team concerning how a clinical are should carry out its work. Organisational culture also reflects the level of acceptable power that is held by the leader.

Power Distance is the team used to describe the level of power a leader exerts over his or her followers.

This level of acceptable power leader has in a team is also variable across international boundaries. Hofstede (1981) identified in his research that different countries hold various acceptable power distances at work.

Countries with greater power distances (Autocracy)	Countries with mid range power distances (Democracy)	Countries with smaller power distances (Laissez-Faire)
• France	• Britain	• Denmark
• Italy	• USA	• Sweden
• Mexico	• Canada	• Austria
• Brazil	• Netherlands	• Israel
• Hong Kong		• New Zealand

Figure 2.3 Global Comparisons of Power Distance
From Hofstede, G. (1980), copyright Geert Hofstede, reproduced with permission

Your own personal style of decision-making in practice will therefore be influenced by the culture of the clinical area you are working in and even when you are practising in the world. Creative decision-making will often allow for more innovative solutions whereas more analytical will use more tried and tested solutions.

- Try the quiz (Table 2.1) to test out which end of the analytical or creative continuum you are.

Table 2.1 Creative or analytical test

	Creative or analytical	Tick	Score
1	I like to think about ideas		
2	I do not like innovative managers		
3	I like organisational traditions		
4	I do not really like change		
5	I really need regular change in my life		
6	I like an ordered environment without too many disruptions		
7	I like people to say what they want freely		
8	I encourage risk taking		
9	I value creativity		
10	I am really a complacent person		
11	I like taking risks		

Table 2.1 (continued)

	Creative or analytical	Tick	Score
12	Other people seem to be more creative than I am		
13	I miss opportunities quite often		
14	I get quite embarrassed when I make mistakes		
15	I give up easily when I can't find a clear solution to a problem		
16	I persist with jobs that need doing		
17	I find difficulty generating ideas		
18	I like to find new solutions to problems		
19	I try to learn from my mistakes		
20	I hate uncertainty		

Give yourself 10 points for each of the following if you ticked them: 1, 4, 5, 7, 8, 9, 11, 16, 18 and 19.

- If you scored less than 70 you are on the more analytical end of the continuum.
- If you scored above 70 you are more creative.

This quiz helps you to look at yourself not only in the way you think but in relation to other people. Some people always seem more ready to take risks and are always doing something new. Other people do not appear to make any great changes to their life. Jill knew a nurse in the 1970s who was horrified at the thought of trying anything other than a regular meat-and-two-vegetable dinner, whereas many of the work group loved to try a curry, a lasagne, a Balti or even get a Chinese take away – in fact, anything for a change. However, life would be very peculiar if we were all the same. Too much creativity in an organisation may lead to insecurity. We need some to be innovators, some to maintain the status quo and some to be resisters to put on the brakes when the pace of change is too rapid (Chapter 9).

Nurses and health care workers, however, do have to think about who to involve in the process of problem solving and decision making and how to involve them. Some helpful ways to think about how to involve people in the stages of problem solving and find a suitable solution can be seen in the following box.

Possible solutions for involving people in problem solving

The five Cs:	The six Is:
Consider	Identify
Consult	Isolate
Commit	Involve
Communicate	Investigate
Check	Implement
	Inquire
Adapted from The Industrial Society (1993)	Adapted from Stott and Walker (1990)

Group think

However, caution must be taken when involving groups of people in identifying problems and solutions. Janis (1968) identified that when groups of people make decisions they are more likely to conform to the majority decision because they do not feel comfortable being an 'outsider'. This has the outcome that less creative solutions may be offered up.

Approaches to problem solving

It has generally been accepted in the *rational approach* that there are stages to problem solving that may help us to understand the concept. Marquis and Huston (1994) illustrate a more traditional problem-solving model.

Traditional problem-solving process

- identify the problem
- gather data to identify cause and consequence
- explore alternative solutions
- evaluate solutions
- select appropriate solution
- implement
- evaluate

This process seems like a useful way of logically looking at problems, but it must be said again that human minds do not always work in such a logical fashion. We do not always work out solutions in a seven-step process. We may look at any of these steps and go steadily round in circles with more complex problems. However, this traditional problem-solving approach is useful in order to see some of the elements involved. Indeed, this approach has been modified to a four-stage process and utilised as the Nursing or Health Visiting Process in addressing the needs and problems of our patients/clients. Midwifery does not have a named midwifery process because most of their clients and patients are undergoing normal physiological changes during pregnancy and childbirth.

Using a broader view allowing for a more creative approach, Simon (1977) and VanGundy (1988) both proposed a three-stage problem-solving process which have similar stages and can be seen in Table 2.2. These two models allow for a broadening of ideas and then a focusing on solutions. The definitions of these can be seen in Table 2.3.

Table 2.2 Problem solving

Simon's Process (1977)	VanGundy's Process (1988)
Intelligence	Problem analysis and redefinition
Design	Idea generation
Choice	Idea evaluation and selection

Table 2.3 Useful problem solving definitions

Intelligence or problem analysis: involves gathering information, analysing it and narrowing it down to a workable problem.

Design or idea generation: involves generating many ideas for courses of action.

Choice or idea evaluation and selection: involves narrowing the courses of action down to a few and then selecting on a basis of set criteria.

Intelligence or problem analysis

As stated earlier, there are a variety of problems from simple to more complex ones. There are lots of problems facing nurses and health care professionals on an hourly basis, which are dealt with quickly and intuitively because the solutions are clear. One way of looking at problems is to define what have been termed 'hard' or 'soft' problems. The characteristics of the two types are seen in Table 2.4

Ackoff (1981) described the hard problems as difficulties and the more complex ones are referred to as 'messy problems' as there is uncertainty and there are no straightforward answers. It is all too easy to try to solve messy problems quickly, like simple problems, without really thinking what the real problem is all about. Hard problems have been defined as having definite

Table 2.4 Problem types

Hard problems or difficulties	Soft messy problems
One clear problem	Complex problem
One clear solution	No one clear solution
Know what needs to be done	Answer can be one of many
Clear methods for working out solution	Uncertainly about the problem
Problem is structured	No obvious way of working it out
	Problem is unstructured

boundaries and soft messy ones as being unbounded (Figure 2.4). Ackoff (1981) felt that there was a need to use many different approaches when dealing with messy problems.

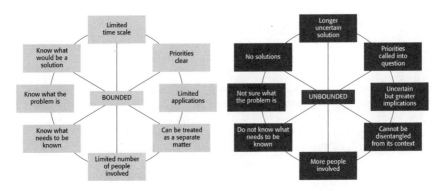

Figure 2.4 Ackoff's bounded/unbounded problems
Adapted from Ackoff (1981)

Try to identify a hard and a soft problem you have encountered in the last week.

Lesley noted that she had a car problem. She bought a new radiator and everything is now fine. This could be seen as a hard problem. For complicated messy problems, it is important that adequate information is gathered about the problem itself. It was Armstrong (1990) who utilised Rudyard Kipling's thoughts on analysing problems:

I keep six honest serving men
(They taught me all I knew)
Their names are What and Why and When
And How and Where and Who

(*The Elephant's Child*, Rudyard Kipling 1902)

This idea of asking questions around the initial symptoms is a very useful way of analysing a problem in more depth. It is also a useful framework when trying to write an assignment to broaden your ideas.

Problem-solving kit

Who, what, where, why, when, how?

- Ask *who* is involved.
- Ask *what* and *where* is the problem.
- *Why* has the problem arisen?
- *When* did it first become a problem and when does it need to be solved?
- Ask *how* the problem came to be noticed and where does it affect.
- Ask *what* are the consequences.

Checkland (1981, p. 316) identified the idea of a real-world problem as 'A problem which arises in the everyday world of events and ideas, and may be perceived differently by different people.'

So it is important to identify who are the problem owners to start with, so that they can help with the other questions of what, when, why and how.

Go back to our original Elfin Ward problem and your thoughts that you wrote down. Did you start to *analyse the problem*? Did you ask yourself *why* the problem arose and *how* it came about and *the various people involved* with the problem?

Thinking back to Elfin Ward, write down some of the issues that require consideration in analysing the problem.

1 Define the problem..
2 How long has it been a problem?...
3 Who is involved?...
4 Why are they involved?..
5 How are they involved?..
6 What are the causes of the problem?......................................
7 What are the possible solutions?..
8 What would be the consequences of each of these solutions?...............
9 When does a decision need to be made?...................................
10 What would help? ....
11 What would hinder? ....
12 What could the consequence be if the problem is not addressed....?

Sister Jenkins had solved an immediate difficulty by getting in agency staff but she needed to look at the whole problem of staff sickness in the long term and the reluctance of both ward and bank staff to cover. Sister Jenkins suspected there was a deeper problem of low staff morale, heavy workloads, lack of recognition and staff conflict. This problem affected her ward staff, other ward staff, bank and agency staff, hospital management and ultimately the whole community that the hospital served. This was an important step in attempting to solve the problem. Her *decisions* were short term and did not really address the root of the problem in the medium to long term. Sister Jenkins then had to start to set an overall aim of improving staff conditions with objectives of raising staff morale, improving staff relationships through team building and introducing a staff development programme. She pencilled into the ward diary a staff meeting to encourage staff to look at the problem together.

Design or idea generation

After examining the problem there is a need to generate ideas in order to look for a solution. The problem owner(s) should be looking at the realistic overall goal in order to start the solution process.

> On Elfin Ward, for example, the problem could be seen to be that of poor staff morale with an underlying problem of poor staff management. The problem owners may set a goal to improve staff relations through training and development.

There are a wide variety of management techniques that can be used to look at complex, messy problems and try to make sense of them. The following techniques may be useful to *generate* a wide range of ideas:

Brainstorming or brainwriting

These techniques are often used in education. They involve asking individuals or groups of individuals to generate ideas around a topic. All ideas are accepted. Brainstorming ideas may be gathered from one individual, from a group of individuals who are physically separated or from a group who are in the same location. The ideas may be generated in the written (brainwriting) or the oral form. Ideas may be shared or not, and ideas may be discussed or not, depending on the organiser. It is a useful way to raise new and varied views on problems. You may choose either brainstorming or brainwriting in the circumstances shown in Table 2.5.

Table 2.5 Brainstorming versus brainwriting

Brainstorming	Brainwriting
1. A small number of people involved.	1. Large number of people involved.
2. Enough time to discuss ideas.	2. Little time to discuss ideas.
3. The status of individuals is similar.	3. Status of indivduals needs to be equalised.

The following techniques are based on the art of diagramming in order to represent the complexities of the issues.

- **Mind mapping:** This starts off with one idea in the centre and, through word association, other ideas are generated from the initial idea to the outside of the diagram. It need not be a systematic process but can be worked in towards the centre as well. A fishbone diagram is sometimes used to illustrate the parts of a whole (see Figure 2.5).

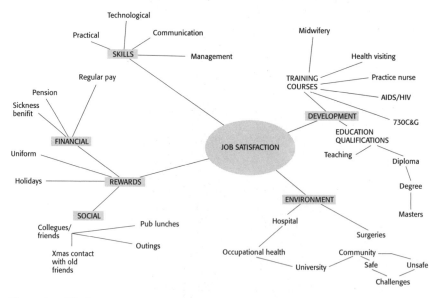

Figure 2.5 Mind map

- **Systems mapping:** Systems mapping involves producing a diagram to show the components within a bounded system (Figure 2.6). This helps us to see the overall relationship between the different parts of a whole.
- **Input-output diagrams:** This is a simple block diagram to show a 'system' with arrows identifying inputs and outputs of the system (Figure 2.7).

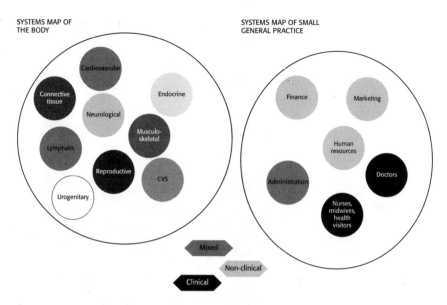

Figure 2.6 Examples of systems maps

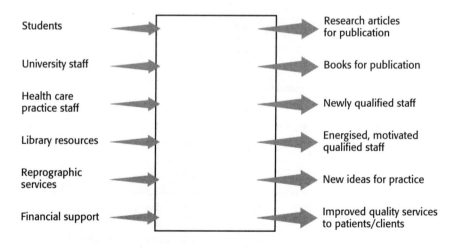

Figure 2.7 Input/output of health care education

- **Flow process diagrams:** This block diagram shows the processes around a system. It may include services, materials or information (Figure 2.8).
- **Critical pathways:** These have been used widely in nursing and medicine to show the 'way through' to an expected end of care (Figure 2.9).

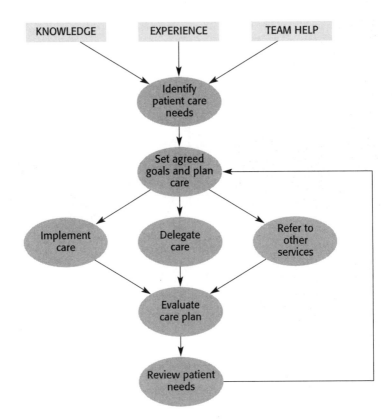

Figure 2.8 Flow process of patient care

- **Control loop:** These are flow diagrams which illustrate the 'feedback mechanism' that controls some of the processes. This is useful in health care to highlight quality audit processes (Figure 2.10).
- **Relationship diagram:** Relationship diagrams are useful tools to illustrate complex relationships within an organisation or even a family. These are often used in community and family nursing (Figure 2.11).

These are just a few of many techniques for generating ideas. There are many other techniques that can be used when very creative ideas are required but those outlined will provide a good basis. VanGundy (1988) provides ample opportunities to explore further techniques.

Patient details				Admission date / Discharge date			Hospital/ward details		
Goals	Assessment consultation	Investigations	Patient activity	Clinical activity	Medication	Diet and hydration	Psycho/social support	Communication education	Discharge
ADMISSION • Patient discusses understanding of pre- & post operative process • Patient is shown to bed and surroundings • Informed consent obtained • Admission assessment, observations and procedures are complete	• Check medical questionnaire • Nursing assessment • Seen by consultant to obtain informed consent • Seen by anaesthetist • Review risk assessment • Physio visit to patient	• FBC • Group and save • ECG • CXR	• Normal activity as mobility allows	• Baseline observations • BP • Pulse • Temp. • ID bracelet • Allergy bracelet Physio teaches • breathing exercises • circulation exercises • supported cough • safe transfer	• Confirm current medication charted by RMO • Patient's own medication stored safely • Anticoagulant therapy prescribed	• Discuss normal habits • Nil by mouth from .... • Inform catering of special diets	• Named nurse explains role and establishes rapport • Identify and alleviate any fears	• Explain about operation and specific post-op care • Initial bed rest • Understanding of catheter • Physio will provide hysterectomy information and discuss	• Discharge plan formulated with patient and family • Anticipated length of stay .... days • Confirm transport arrangements
Signature AM									
PM									
Night									

Figure 2.9 Example of care pathway (hysterectomy)

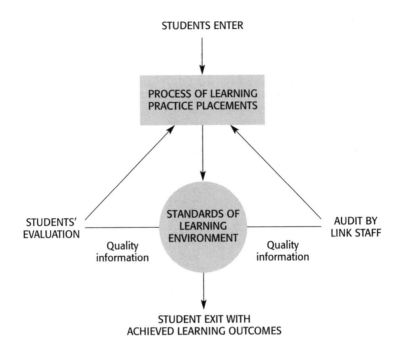

Figure 2.10 Control loop system for practice placements

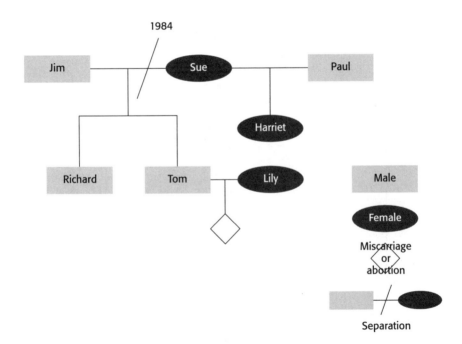

Figure 2.11 Relationships diagram in family nursing

Choice or idea evaluation and selection

Once a range of ideas for tackling a problem has been identified, the next stage is to narrow it down into a choice for a decision to be made. It was Simon (1977) who differentiated between ideal and real decision making. He noted that many models highlighted a rational and logical approach but that in reality men and women were rarely rational and logical. He identified the two types of decision making based on an 'economic person' or an 'administrative person'. The economic person set objectives and goals and their solutions were aimed at *maximising* the benefits whereas the administrative person was more of a realistic decision maker and aimed to reach *satisfaction* rather than *maximisation* (Table 2.6).

Table 2.6 'The economic person' versus 'the administrative person'

Economic	Administrative
Decide in a rational manner	Make 'good enough' decisions
Complete knowledge of problem	Incomplete fragmented knowledge
Complete list of possible alternatives	Difficult to predict the future consequences of alternatives
Rational system of preferences	Decision from small choice of alternatives
Select decision for maximum results	Select decision based on 'satisfying'

Initially, our Sister Jenkins made a 'satisfaction' decision but when she realised the complexity of the problem she started to aim for 'maximisation' when she set out an agenda for involving the whole team. Decision making relies on determining the consequences and constraints of the available choices. When dealing with clinical decisions, the importance of interpersonal skills in observation and communication is vital. Nursing assessment and 'diagnosis' rely on good decision making for planning care. The North American Nursing Diagnosis Association (NANDA) defines a nursing diagnosis as 'a clinical judgement about an individual, family or community response to actual or potential health problems/life processes which provides the basis for defining therapy toward achievement of outcomes for which the nurse is accountable' (Carpenito 1991 p. 65).

In terms of decision making in nursing, midwifery and health visiting, there have been some interesting ideas raised. Benner (1984) argued that expert practitioners viewed situations holistically, drawing on past, concrete experiences, whereas those at the competent or proficient level had to use conscious problem solving. Expert professional judgement relies on intuitive skills. Marsden (1998) in her study of decision making in casualty, identified that intuition (as a skill) was based on a collection of experiences of similar clinical presentations, expertise, good questioning and good decision making. Questioning skills were thus seen as critical to expert decision making. However, researching decision making in nurses, midwives and health visitors is notoriously difficult. Lemmer (1998) set out to look at decision making in health visiting and identified the need for more research because 'the implementation of the NHS reforms has led to an increasing emphasis upon the need for analytical thinking'. This may be seen as being at the expense of intuitive thinking. He goes on to highlight that the value of intuitive reasoning in health visiting may be lost at the expense of analytical thinking. The use of intuition and interpersonal skills is recognised as a valid subject in health care education (Schon 1983, Benner 1984). However, Lemmer noted that the methods and skills for decision making are rarely addressed during training and development. It could be said, though, that decision making on ethical issues is usually included as an important part of most courses now. The many dilemmas that face nurses, midwives and health visitors, such as abortion, euthanasia and health care rationing, show that students need to identify the range of perspectives and ethical principles to make choices of involvement. Problem solving and decision making are skills that will develop throughout your career. You will get better at knowing what to do in an emergency and in caring for people. You will also learn how to take opportunities and risks for your future development. You may move into new demanding positions or, on the other hand, you may not get jobs you really wanted. You will make mistakes but do not think that you are ever alone. We all make mistakes but the important aspect of this chapter is that we learn to manage our problems and that we do not offend too many people on the way. We also need to try to forgive those that make mistakes that affect us because they too are learning.

1 Identify two approaches to problem solving.
2 Discuss the differences between the two.
3 Try to remember three aspects of problem solving that will affect how you think about yourself as a problem solver.
4 When you next get an assignment that causes you concern, try to utilise any of the techniques to broaden your ideas.

Conclusion

This chapter has given you an overview of the role of problem solving and decision making in clinical practice. The main approaches in this area have been highlighted and have reflected the various problem-solving characteristics that might be evident. Practical examples of idea generation techniques have been given in order to help you with complex problems that may be encountered in health care.

WITHDRAWN

Summary of key points

This chapter has looked at the various aspects of problem solving and decision making.

- **Problem solving:** Relates to finding a solution for a perceived difficulty in a situation.

- **Decision making:** Is part of problem solving, it is a response to a set of criteria requiring a solution, i.e. choosing the 'best fit'.

- **Problem solvers:** Are people who are involved, through rank, knowledge, opportunity or power base, to look for solutions.

- **Problem owners:** Are those people who are affected by the difficulty or the solutions.

- **Intelligence:** Is about a higher order of knowledge.

- **Idea generation:** Is the process through which a breadth of ideas is created.

- **Idea evaluation:** Is assessing the effect of the chosen idea based on a set of criteria.

References

Ackoff R L (1981) The art and science of mess management, in Mabey C and Mayonwhite B (eds)) (1993) *Managing Change* (2nd edn) Paul Chapman, Open University, pp. 47–54

Armstrong M (1990) *How To Be an Even Better Manager*, Kogan Page

Benner P (1984) *From Novice to Expert: Excellence in Power in Clinical Nursing Practice*, Jossey-Bass

Carpenito L (1991) The NANDA definition of nursing diagnosis, in Carroll-Johnson R M (ed.) (1991) *Classification of Nursing Diagnoses: Proceedings of the Ninth Conference*, Lippincott

Checkland, P B (1981) *Systems Thinking, Systems Practice*, John Wiley

Drucker P (1964) *Managing for Results*, Pan Books

Hamm R M (1988) cited by Luker K, Hogg C, Austin L, Ferguson B and Smith K (1998) Decision Making: the context of nurse prescribing, *Journal of Advanced Nursing* **27**, 657–65

Hofstede G (1980) Culture's consequences: *International difference in work related values*, Sage

Janis I L (1968) *Victims of Group Think: A Psychological Study of Foreign Policy Decisions and Fiascos*, Houghton Mifflin

Lemmer W E (1998) Successive surveys of an expert panel: research into decision making with health visitors, *Journal of Advanced Nursing* **27**, 538–45

Marquis B and Huston C (1994) *Management Decision Making for Nurses*, Lippincott

Marsden J (1998) Decision-making in A & E by expert nurses, *Nursing Times* **94** (41)

Schon D A (1983) *The Reflective Practitioner: How Professionals Think in Action*, Basic Books

Simon H A (1977) *The New Science of Management Decision* (revised edn) Prentice Hall

Stewart R (1989) *Leading in the NHS: A Practical Guide*, Macmillan

Stewart R (1996) *Leading in the NHS: A Practical Guide* (2nd edn), Macmillan

Stott K and Walker A (1990) *Making Management Work: A Practical Approach*, Prentice Hall

The Industrial Society (1993) *Management Skills: A Practical Handbook*, The Industrial Society

VanGundy A B (1988) *Techniques of Structured Problem Solving* (2nd edn) Van Nostrand Reinhold

Vroom V and Yetton P (1973) *Leadership and Decision Making*, University of Pittsburgh Press

Further reading

Adair J (1971) *Training for Decisions*, Gower

Adair J (1985) *Effective Decision Making*, Pan Books

Carnevali D and Thomas M D (1993) *Diagnostic Reasoning and Treatment Decision Making in Nursing*, Lippincott

Cooke S and Slack N (1991) *Making Management Decisions* (2nd edn) Prentice Hall

Handy C (1991) *Gods of Management*, Century Business

Hurst K (1993) *Problem Solving in Nursing Practice*, Scutari Press

Leigh A (1993) *Decisions Decisions*, Institute of Personnel Management

3

Getting your message across

By the end of this chapter you will have had the opportunity to:

- recognise the importance of effective communication strategies
- distinguish between formal and informal communication networks
- identify various forms of formal communication in health care
- recognise the purpose and context of formal communication
- discuss the importance of quality record keeping
- discuss the changing context of formal communication in health care
- discuss the advantages and disadvantages of networking.

Introduction

In the last two chapters you have been asked to examine the image you project to others, the way you organise your time, and the way in which you might solve problems and make decisions. This chapter will now go on to look at communication skills and how you get your message or point of view across to others, recognising that this is a two-way process whereby you can learn as much from colleagues as they learn from you. By talking to others, forming networks, coalitions and alliances you can develop professional power. Professional power may be seen in many guises and situations but in all cases it has the potential ability to get things done in order to achieve goals. Effective communication is vital in any employment and nowhere is it so important as in the delivery of care. Indeed, Harvey (1997) noted that communication was at the top of the list of most important skills required by potential employers, closely followed by team working and interpersonal skills. There are many ways to communicate, e.g. formal/informal; verbal/non-verbal; written/electronic; face to face; sign/braille, all of which have their part to play. Within this chapter there will be discussion related to formal and informal communication networks together with their effective use within the workplace, following which there will be an examination of networking and its benefits.

Models of communication

A model may set out to describe the process and stages through which someone or something has to pass in order to achieve a specified aim. It also acts as a checklist to ensure that each stage has been negotiated successfully. The basic communications model takes the form of a chain of events (Figure 3.1) comprising:

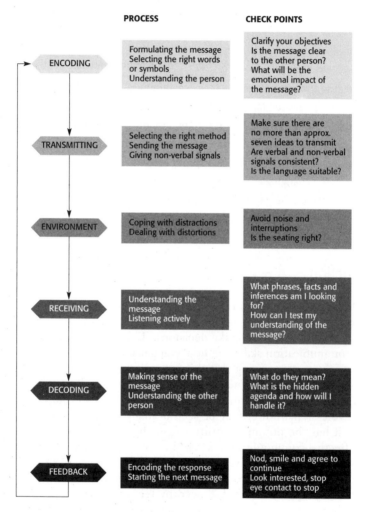

PROCESS	CHECK POINTS
ENCODING — Formulating the message Selecting the right words or symbols Understanding the person	Clarify your objectives Is the message clear to the other person? What will be the emotional impact of the message?
TRANSMITTING — Selecting the right method Sending the message Giving non-verbal signals	Make sure there are no more than approx. seven ideas to transmit Are verbal and non-verbal signals consistent? Is the language suitable?
ENVIRONMENT — Coping with distractions Dealing with distortions	Avoid noise and interruptions Is the seating right?
RECEIVING — Understanding the message Listening actively	What phrases, facts and inferences am I looking for? How can I test my understanding of the message?
DECODING — Making sense of the message Understanding the other person	What do they mean? What is the hidden agenda and how will I handle it?
FEEDBACK — Encoding the response Starting the next message	Nod, smile and agree to continue Look interested, stop eye contact to stop

Figure 3.1 The basic communications model
Adapted from Weightman (1999)

- encoding
- transmitting
- environment
- receiving
- decoding
- feedback.

Problems may occur at any of these points so it is worth working out where the problem might originate so that it might be addressed. This is applicable within all individual or group interactions, across whole departments, within your working life and within your personal life. So what is the purpose of communication?

- Think back over the last 24 hours.
- Make a note of what you did and how much of this time was spent in contact with someone else.
- What purpose did the communication serve?

You might have thought of many reasons to communicate with others and they could have included some or all of the following:

- to get something
- to try to change someone's behaviour (innovation)
- to find out about something
- to sort out a problem and raise motivation (integration)
- to express your feelings about someone or something
- to ensure that everyone gets the same message (regulation)
- to give factual information that people need to proceed efficiently with their work (Weightman 1999).

The list could go on but whatever the situation you can be sure that you used the chain of communication events depicted in Figure 3.1. Overall the purpose of communication is to ensure that messages are received and understood in order to make life easier both in working and home environments. Of course the system goes 'pear-shaped' at times and communication is not as effective as it could be but if we understand what is happening then we can do something about it.

Formal communication

Formal communication in nursing is an important aspect of all care delivery. All nurses need to be aware of the skills and knowledge needed for effective communication and how to communicate with other members of the multi-disciplinary and multi-agency teams effectively. Poor communication can lead to poor continuing care and, at its worst, incompetent practice leading to fatal errors with resulting disciplinary action. Learning to be an effective and professional communicator is often seen as a difficult journey.

Write down what you think are your strengths and weaknesses in communication.

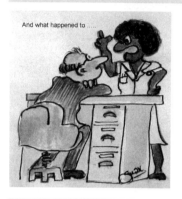

Jill is not good at telephoning friends and family on a regular basis. This is probably due to the amount of telephoning and talking that she does on a daily basis at work. She also needs to work on her listening skills as she feels she can voice her own opinions without any problem and she always has to think about asking others for their views.

Types of formal communication

There are numerous types of formal communication channels in health care. Formal communication involves formal pieces of information that can be used to convey ideas and feelings to other people, in order to influence them in some way. In health care, records of professional views and actions are filed in patient/client notes or are kept for formal occasions such as meetings or ultimately may be used in court.

Can you name some examples of formal communication you have come across recently?

You may have thought about the following: care records, reports, letters, interviews for a job or a student place, memos, articles for publication, research. Most of these will only be described in the context of health care as not all those in practice will be expected to use these forms of communication but record keeping will be highlighted as a vital and important aspect of health care provision for all practitioners.

Purpose of formal records

There are four main reasons that we formally communicate with other people:

1. To inform.
2. To instruct.
3. To motivate.
4. To seek information.

When we do this in health care, it should really be seen in the context of the core business of providing quality nursing, midwifery or health visiting care.

Formal care records

Lumby (1991) notes that caring has its communication roots built on an oral tradition. This has meant that early nursing knowledge was not recognised or even regarded as credible. This tradition has meant that it has not even been possible to collect nursing and health care practice knowledge books as it was doctors who always published medical and care books. Nursing and midwifery knowledge was seen as being of lesser value than medicine and merely a part of it. O'Brien and Pearson (1993) suggest that there are two reasons that real knowledge of nursing practice is seldom documented:

1. Nursing information is central to practice and is taken for granted and accepted by expert nurses almost 'without thinking'.
2. Such forms of knowledge fall outside what is deemed to be real science.

It is interesting to note that Florence Nightingale (1859) felt that writing down one's observations about patients was a mental crutch that would diminish the nurse's capacity to observe and remember. She permitted it reluctantly, 'but if you cannot get the habit of observation one way or another, you had better give up being a nurse, for it is not your calling, however kind and anxious you may be' (cited in Eggland and Heinemann 1994, p. 4).

The oral tradition was useful where nursing was simple but as the hospitals grew, shift duty was required, health need awareness expanded and written channels were legally required to pass information on to different staff. Eggland and Heinemann (1994) define a clinical record as 'The comprehensive collection of data that describes a patient's condition, health care needs, health care services received and responses to care'.

In the light of what was said earlier, what do you think is the purpose(s) of health care records?

They are generally used to inform others of the needs and progress of patients, clients and families in respect of their overall health. However, they are also used to instruct others of what is expected of them in continuing care. When used with patients/clients they can also motivate and help in the learning process. They are also useful learning and motivational aids for students and learners and therefore we aim to keep them focused on 'best practice'.

The kardex was a system that was introduced to support a verbal 'handover' in a ward office. In the 1980s when the nursing process was being introduced, further systems were required to bring in nursing care plans. In true bureaucratic NHS style, more paper records were felt to be required rather than streamlining the process of care record keeping. In many areas still, there are duplicated records that mean that nurses' time in patient contact is lost at the expense of administration.

> Can you reflect on a clinical area you have visited recently and identify whether you felt there were good examples of record keeping or ones that were confusing or badly kept?

Nursing and health care is now more diverse than ever. This diversity stretches over day surgery, medium-stay surgical, continuing care in nursing homes, outpatient departments, practice nursing, midwifery, district nursing, accident and emergency and theatre nursing as well as health visiting and school nursing. This means that record keeping will be adapted to meet the needs of the environment. Hour-by-hour recording will not be as commonplace in nursing homes as it will perhaps be in theatres.

There are a variety of records available in health care.

> Can you think of the various types of patient records that may be seen in health care?

You may have thought about the following types: hand-written, patient-held, critical pathways, computerised, multi-agency. You may not have seen all these examples but look out for them in the future.

> What do you think are the advantages and disadvantages of computerised care records?

You may have felt that they are more efficient in saving time for documenting usual and expected aspects of care. They may also be used to specify aspects of practice expected in certain care situations. The use of computerised records can also save space in GP surgeries where the problem of storage over many years is problematic. The disadvantages are that the individuality of care is not reflected in the documentation and that there is an inability or difficulty in highlighting specific issues for individuals. Doctors sometimes complain that some of their computerised records do not allow them to document certain areas they have checked to be normal, when they perform a clinical examination. It will only allow them to register a problem. There are also fears that computerised records may be 'lost' if the hardware is stolen or breaks down for a period of time. So in many areas both manual and computerised records are kept simultaneously.

Record keeping and the law

Another important aspect to note is that record keeping is seen in the context of professional standards of practice and within a legal framework. There are ethical issues concerning the following:

- integrity
- truth
- respect
- confidentiality
- consent, and
- informed decision making.

The importance for documentation in future will grow as the culture of litigation appears to be on the increase and health care expectations rise. So much for Nightingale's view!

Value of record keeping

Record keeping is not only used as a form of communication but can be used for the following:

- legal protection
- reimbursement
- patient education
- quality assurance
- research.

Records and documentation are the primary communication tool that reflects nursing and care philosophies, models, structure, processes and outcomes. Nurses, midwives and health visitors communicate with each other and other agencies through their records by:

- collection of data to identify needs
- problems and concerns
- reactions and responses to existing or potential health needs
- goals set and planned interventions
- review and goal evaluation which should highlight the effectiveness of the professional input by examining the outcomes or responses.

It is also important to note what health care services have been offered to clients as they may have been refused through choice. The UKCC (1998) provides new guidelines for professional record keeping; the updated version now clarifies issues and stresses the importance of professional practice. It sets out the need for the following:

- facts, consistency and accuracy
- current information on care and condition of patient/client
- written clearly in a manner such that the text cannot be erased
- dated, timed and signed
- not to include abbreviations, jargon, meaningless phrases, irrelevant speculation and offensive subjective statements
- readable on any photocopies
- written wherever possible with the involvement of the patient/client and their carer.

The Access to Health Record Act 1990 and the Data Protection Act 1984 give patients and clients specific rights concerning their records (Table 3.1). Nursing and health care record keeping has been criticised recently (Castledine 1998, Tingle 1998). The deterioration in record keeping is thought to be due to various factors:

- record keeping is not thought to be a skill that is taught and corrected when poor
- complexity of personnel giving care and recording in nursing records
- complexity of health care interventions and communication channels.

Table 3.1 Length of storage time for health records

Maternity records	25 years
Children	Up to the age of 25 years/10 years after death
Patients under Mental Health Act (1983)	20 years/10 years after death
Prisoners and armed forces	Not destroyed
Others	10 years

Tingle notes that the Clinical Systems Group (CSG) of the Department of Health wrote a report in 1998, *Improving Clinical Communications*. Their findings showed that:

- few records show *decisions* and *who is responsible* for carrying out tasks
- where care is shared there is rarely a full record of all events, even in GP records
- *specific advice or information* is rarely recorded
- inaccurate information
- widespread duplication.

Why do you think there are these weaknesses?

It would be easy to say that there is never enough time but the main problem lies in the management of the clinical areas. These may be lacking in one or all of the following:

- Patient/client focus;
- Poor training;
- Poor monitoring of records.

Documentation for care therefore needs to be constantly monitored and audited to measure standards and to aim to improve the skills of professional staff in record writing, so giving value to the professional care on offer.

Meetings

These are where groups of people come together for a range of reasons such as problem solving, negotiation, decision making and information sharing. More formal meetings require agendas to be produced prior to the meeting date, and minutes and/or action plans to be sent afterwards. There should be a recognised 'chair' who has the role of timekeeper, agenda manager and sometimes referee. It is also important that the chair introduces everybody and is aware of the problems of power, control and 'group think'. Rules and/or conventions may also guide the more formal meetings.

- Try to attend an RCN/RCM/MSF/UNISON meeting to see how they are organised.
- Write a reflective diary on what you experienced.

There are recognised advantages of face-to-face contact with others in terms of team building but they are often time-consuming and expensive. Having attended many case conferences for child protection, it was obvious to Jill that some members never prepared for the meeting. Sometimes this was frustrating because the meeting had to be adjourned to another date. When you think of a meeting going on for two or three hours and everyone's hourly salary, there is a need for a certain discipline in management. If you need to go to a meeting, be sure to know what possible contribution you can make and if you are unsure, discuss it with a manager or mentor.

Minutes

It is important to keep a record of formal meetings in order to ensure that everyone is aware of what took place and what decisions were made. Minutes should always be read, in order that everyone agrees on the reliability of the record. This is important as content may become policy.

The minutes should contain a record of the following:

- details of meeting place and date
- names of those present
- apologies from those absent
- agreement on the previous minutes
- matters arising
- business items
- date of next meeting
- any other business.

Policies and procedures

Policies are written forms of internal communication to show employees *how* the organisation will achieve its objectives. It is a way of representation of 'the way things are done here'. Policies provide the broad framework for decision making in an organisation, as well as clarifying roles and responsibilities. Mullins (1993, p. 281) states that policy is 'guidelines for organizational action and the implementation of goals and objectives'. However, some policies are guidelines that are directly influenced by government legislation.

- Think about some policies you know about in the health service that fall into this category.
- How do they affect patient/client care?

The ones that first spring to mind, perhaps, are the equal opportunity policies and the health and safety regulations. These are useful policies for valuing all staff in terms of discrimination and personal health and this will ultimately affect patient/client morale. On the other hand, policies could be seen as a way of *controlling* staff (Huczynski and Buchanan 1991, p. 587) and showing staff what is acceptable behaviour and what is not.

Procedures are even more specific written communication about how certain tasks will be carried out. You may have seen procedures about what to do in case of a fire. After reading them, you should then have the knowledge about your responsibility in terms of alerting the fire brigade, making patients safe and evacuating buildings.

- When you are next in practice, identify the whereabouts of the policies and procedures for that clinical area.
- What types of procedures are currently in use?
- How many of the procedures are influenced by evidence and research?

Presentations

In health care, presentations are frequently used in terms of cascading information verbally to a number of people.

Can you think of the advantages and disadvantages of this method of communication?

The advantages may be getting information quickly to a greater number of people. A presentation may also be a forum to change attitudes and values, or may be about information sharing. It is also a good method for self-learning if you have to present a topic. Many of you will recognise the amount of knowledge you acquire when you have to make a presentation in a classroom. The disadvantages are that it involves public speaking skills, and staff may find they have not got the confidence or skills in this area. It does involve releasing staff from their normal day-to-day role and is time-consuming and thus expensive.

Reports

Reports are commonly required in nursing, midwifery and health visiting. A report is a document that may:

- state facts
- analyse issues
- give professional opinions
- report progress
- draw conclusions
- make proposals.

They are commonly used to inform or even persuade others, as well as helping to initiate change. Reports could be written to bid for more resources in a ward or within a team, or when a particular service needs to be evaluated. Reports are useful for presenting an assessment of a patient for a multi-agency case conference in order to provide clarification. They should be factual and written with patients or carers. It is usually up to a senior member of the team to produce a report but they may gather information and opinions from any member of the nursing or midwifery team.

Identify any national reports affecting health care that you may be aware of from your past or present coursework.

Some very old reports that had an impact on nursing were the Salmon Report (Ministry of Health 1966) and the Cumberledge Report (Department of Health and Social Security 1985); more recently 'Changing Childbirth' (1993) and a range of Commission Reports such as 'With Respect to Old Age' (Audit Commission 1999) and 'Seen but not heard' (Audit Commission 1994) are more relevant reports. Reports often precede policy making at all levels.

Reports need to be precise, formal and concise in their style. The third person ('It was found that…') is more commonly used but the first person may also be used. They are usually in a particular format that identifies specific sections of a report. Pages should be numbered and a specific numbering system should be used for paragraphs and subsections for ease in group discussions. The following will be common in reports:

- title page
- summary
- terms of reference
- procedure (for gathering information)
- main body of findings
- conclusions
- recommendations.

The *title page* is usually a front cover with the name of the report, the author, the date and the person or group to whom it is to be sent. The *summary* then comments on the main point of the report, general conclusions and proposals.

Terms of reference are the objectives or expected outcome of the report, for example 'To identify the current health needs of family X', 'To present the views of family X on the needs of their son', 'To propose nursing/midwifery/health visiting input for future optimum health'. The *procedure* identifies the methods for gathering information. The *main body of findings* will analyse what was found in gathering information, following which the *conclusions* will discuss what are believed to be the choices for the future. *Recommendations* will identify any recommended decisions and a practical basis for action. *References* are normally kept to a minimum and *appendices* contain large amounts of details if necessary in order to keep the main body of the report concise. Longer reports may include a contents page and very short reports may have modifications of the above sections.

Letters

Letters are used in a variety of ways in health care: letters of referral, letters for influencing decisions and letters for influencing action. In terms of formality, it is useful to keep copies of letters sent as well as those received to reflect the total correspondence. These copies will help in cases of query at a later date. Nurses, midwives and health visitors are an influential professional group. Their letters in respect of patient health status can make an impact on welfare decisions by other agencies.

Memos

These are almost like quick notes of internal communication and are often used between members in the same organisation. These can become a permanent record of action agreed or actions recommended. Any written communication can be ascribed 'formal' status. They need to be carefully filed. It should be remembered that memos are still considered official documentation, regardless of their limited content.

Informal communication

Informal communication is considered to be the type of regular communication that is not recorded and goes on daily between patients/clients and health care staff as well as between staff groups. Informal communication involves non-verbal and verbal communication. It is evident in ward 'handovers' that a lot more information is passed among staff and students than just patient

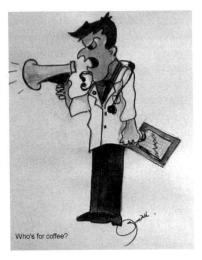

Who's for coffee?

information. There are social exchanges, clarification of terms, requests and responses for support in dealing with difficult events. It is this informal communication that plays an important role in helping new people settle in to the particular culture of the clinical area. It also helps in team building as well as serving as a means of knowledge transfer. Lally (1999) identified in her research into nurse communication in the intershift hand-over, that goals and values relating to nursing practice were passed on to the team, so facilitating team cohesiveness.

What do you think could be the negative aspects of informal communication?

If you have ever been employed as bank or agency staff, the informal communication can actually work against you. You may feel like an outsider if you have not been to the 'night out' or your opinion on a new change is not asked, or, even worse, you have not contributed to the coffee so you are made to feel that you cannot accept a drink. The value of the oral tradition has recently been raised in nursing, midwifery and health visiting with the focus on 'reflective practice' (further discussed in Chapter 4). Thus this oral tradition is changing what may have previously been considered informal communication into a formally accepted method of learning.

Networking

The effective initiation and maintenance of social relationships for career-related purposes are often called *networks*. Networking is about making contacts and connections; the term 'networking' is often used to describe the support system that exists between professionals, organisations and social environments and they take different forms. They may be made up of a variety of members both from within and outside a specific organisation. It may be thought of as the 'I know a man who can' arrangement; similarly, 'you owe me one' is another feature, giving the notion that this is a two-way process of helping and gaining power through knowledge. In order to care effectively, nurses, midwives and health visitors must understand and recognise the importance of power and be ready to accept or use it. Bennis and Nannus (1985) suggest that power is the basic energy required for sustaining action and translating intention into reality.

If we belong to a group, then life becomes much easier, as we will know if ever we are 'sent to Coventry'. The feeling of being 'out of it' is not a nice one; we much prefer the feeling of 'belonging'. We all belong to various groups or networks, which are collective titles for the people and organisations with which we communicate (Barker 1990). Networking can also be used to support people who face obstacles in their careers.

Purposes of networking

The purposes of networking are:

- seeking information related to enhancing patient care (Chapter 5);
- finding a mentor (Chapter 6);
- seeking information related to assignments (Chapter 3);
- seeking information related to prospective employers/employment (Chapters 7;11;12);
- managing change (Chapter 8);
- becoming an effective leader (Chapter 6);
- getting career advice (Chapter 12);
- updating professional skills (Chapter 12).

There is very little literature about networking *per se* but Hamilton and Kiefer (1986) identified four prerequisites to successful networking:

1. Each individual in the network must have a basic self-interest; a desire to improve or get ahead.
2. Each individual must be willing to use other people and be used in return.
3. There must be a balance of power within the networking relationship.
4. Individuals in networking must have a positive self-concept and feel they can contribute to others.

Together with this, it could be said that there are four other elements to be taken into consideration:

1. Social contact (party/meeting).
2. Common interest/attribute.
3. Potential or actual need for contact.
4. Need for contact point for information.

One aspect of networking that is sometimes forgotten is that it involves giving as well as taking. To be involved in social networks means that one can be expected on occasions to offer help, information, support or advice as well as to receive it. For those who find it difficult to consider spending time on entirely altruistic activities, there are two consolations. First, it is possible to learn something useful from other people even if the relationship is more give than take. Second, the social norm of reciprocity means that a favour given now is one that all parties involved can legitimately expect to be repaid at some later date (Gouldner 1960). Conversely, declining to help a person now has obvious negative potential consequences for the future. When considering assessments for your course you might wish to develop a network of like-minded people who will each research a section of the topic; they could then meet together to share the information with others in the study group. However, if this sharing is to do with the preparation of assignments, then the written work *must* be done individually to avoid the pitfalls of plagiarism. In this way a considerable amount of information can be gathered and time used effectively. While it may be hidden, the way in which we accrue information about the best method of delivering care, for example, will be through talking to others, as well as reading the literature, examining the information in relation to the condition of the client/patient, and making informed decisions as to what will be the most effective path to take. Of course the physical writing of any work will be the work of each individual without collusion with others, but considerable time is saved in researching a given topic.

Imagine you need to research new evidence in the subject of catheterisation

- List the ways in which networking might help you in achieving your goal.
- Identify the main members of your network group.
- Is there anyone who is not on your list but, on reflection, you think they should be?

Having identified the main members of your network group for a particular set of circumstances you might now like to consider how they would help you and indeed how you would reciprocate. Sometimes it is about 'pay-back time', 'I helped you before, now it's your turn to help me' or it could be just about 'being there' for a colleague or friend.

It is vital to establish and maintain one's professional reputation (Arthur 1994) within and beyond the people with whom one has contact in day-to-day work. One analysis showed that people in management roles already tend to have larger social networks than others in posts where management was not part of the role (Carroll and Teo 1996). The authors concluded on the basis of survey data from 268 managers and 366 non-managers in the USA that:

> When compared to non-managers, managers' show wider organisational membership networks – they belong to more clubs, societies and the like. Managers also have larger core discussion networks, and these contain more co-workers, more strangers, and more people with whom the focal person has close or intimate ties. (Carroll and Teo 1996, p. 437)

This is in line with the picture of managerial work painted by Mintzberg (1973) and others as being dominated by the making and maintenance of contacts outside the formal organisational chain of command.

The last observation in the extract above is perhaps particularly signifi-cant. It is sometimes argued that managers' contacts tend to be shallow, confined to the task-related needs of the moment, but Carroll and Teo's find-ings suggested otherwise.

Arnold (1997) suggests that there is little doubt that the twenty-first cen-tury will see great emphasis on networking, especially since with the availability of electronic communication, the scope for self-presentation and the range of skills required to do it well are both increasing. More working at home and the blurring of organisational boundaries mean that your achieve-ments and experiences may be less obvious to other people; telephone, fax and e-mail communication take on greater importance. For some people their work is fairly open to scrutiny and social networks that cross organisa-tional boundaries are relatively well formed. Also, for some people the formation of close friendships may override the need for impression manage-ment. You know you can safely be candid about your weaknesses when you are with your really good friends.

Conclusion

Throughout this chapter you have been examining a variety of ways in which you can communicate both formally and informally, some of the legal aspects of communication together with the need for maintaining effective health care records. The model of communication depicted described the process and stages of effective communication. Following this we examined the effect of formal communication on effective care delivery by itemising its types, purpose, types of record, the law related to this activity and the overall value of record keeping. Informal communication is equally important, as is net-working. The feeling of 'belonging' to others helps with coping. Having examined these factors we are now able to move on and use them in consid-ering role expectations within the next chapter.

Summary of key points

This chapter has examined the following areas:

- **Models of communication**: Examined the chain of events for effective com-munication.

- **Formal communication**: Looked at individual strengths and weaknesses in communication, their effects on patient care and the legal implications of effective record keeping.

- **Informal communication**: Examined the art of networking and its effect on patient care together with its effect on personal growth.

References

Arnold J (1997) *Managing Careers into the 21st Century*, Paul Chapman

Arthur M B (1994) The boundaryless career: a new perspective for organisational enquiry, *Journal of Organisational Behaviour*, vol. 15, pp. 259–306, cited in Arnold (1997)

Audit Commission (1994) *Seen but not heard: Co-ordinating Community Child Health and Social Services for Children in Need*, HMSO

Audit Commission (1999) *With Respect to Old Age*, HMSO

Barker P (1990) Professional networking, cited in Cormack D F S (ed.) (1990) *Developing Your Career in Nursing*, Chapman & Hall

Bennis W and Nannus B (1985) *Leaders*, Harper and Row

Carroll G R and Teo A C (1996) On social networks of managers, *Academy of Management Journal*, vol. 39, pp. 421–40, cited in Arnold (1997)

Castledine G (1998) The blunders found in nursing documentation, *British Journal of Nursing* **7**(19), 1218

Clinical Systems Group (1998) *Improving Clinical Communications*, Two Ten Communications

Department of Health (1993) *Changing Childbirth*, HMSO

Department of Health and Social Security (1985) *Neighbourhood Nursing (Chair Julia Cumberledge)*, HMSO

Eggland E and Heinemann D (1994) *Nursing documentation: Charting, Recording and Reporting*, Lippincott

Gouldner A W (1960) The norm of reciprocity: a preliminary statement, *American Sociological Review*, vol. 25, pp. 161–78 cited in Arnold (1997)

Hamilton J M and Kiefer M E (1986) *Survival Skills for the New Nurse*, Lippincott, cited in Marquis B L and Huston C J (1992) *Leadership Roles and Management Functions in Nursing* (2nd edn) Lippincott

Harvey L (1997) *Report to Association of Graduate Recruiters*, Warwick University, 7–9 July

Huczynski A and Buchanan D (1991) *Organizational Behaviour* (2nd edn) Prentice Hall

Lally S (1999) An investigation into the functions of nurses' communication at the inter-shift handover, *Journal of Nursing Management*, **7**, 29–36

Lumby J (1991) Threads of an emerging discipline, in Gray G and Pratt R (eds) (1991) *Towards a Discipline of Nursing*, Churchill Livingstone

Ministry of Health, British Home and Health Department (1966) *Report of the Committee on Senior Nursing Staff Structure (Chair Brian Salmon)*, HMSO

Mintzberg H (1973) *The Nature of Managerial Work*, Harper and Row

Mullins L J (1993) *Management and Organisational Behaviour* (3rd edn) Pitman

O'Brien B and Pearson A (1993) Unwritten knowledge in nursing: consider the spoken as well as the written word, *Scholarly Inquiry for Nursing Practice* **7** (2), 111–124

Tingle J (1998) Nurses must improve their record keeping skills, *British Journal of Nursing* **7**, 245

UKCC (1998) *Guidelines for Records and Record keeping*, UKCC

Weightman J (1999) *Introducing Organisational Behaviour*, Addison Wesley Longman

Further reading

Castledine G (1994) The standard of nursing records should be raised, *British Journal of Nursing* **7**(3), 172

Cormack D F S (ed.) (1990) *Developing your Career in Nursing*, Chapman and Hall

Department of Health and Social Security (1983) *NHS Management Enquiry (Chair R Griffiths)*, HMSO

Iles V (1997) *Really Managing Health Care*, Open University Press

Feldman D C and Klich N (1991) Impression management and career strategies, cited in Arnold (1997)

Marquis B L and Huston C J (1992) *Leadership Roles and Management Functions in Nursing*, (2nd edn) Lippincott

Mullins L J (1999) *Management and Organisational Behaviour* (5th edn) Pitman Publishing

Sullivan E J and Decker P J (1997) *Effective Leadership and Management in Nursing* (4th edn) Addison-Wesley

4 ~~WITHDRAWN~~

Role expectations

By the end of this chapter you will have had the opportunity to:

- discuss differing role expectations within the health care environment
- define the role of the student and the newly qualified practitioner
- identify the qualities required by the practitioner when managing for the first time
- define professional accountability and responsibility
- discuss the effects of the Professional Code of Conduct on practice
- recognise the need for effective use of reflective practice.

Introduction

The first four chapters have examined the individual's traits in terms of their ability to get organised, make decisions effectively and communicate with others. Within the final chapter of this section we will examine the work of an individual practitioner. We will attempt to explain the role expectations you may have and see how those expectations may become reality.

It is always useful to have a role model. It is difficult to define a role model but theorists suggest that modelling one's behaviour on others is an important way of learning and it does seem that in this context 'actions speak louder than words'. As you go through your education and training you will see others working in a way you would want to emulate and this helps to colour your picture of what the student or newly qualified nurse, midwife or health visitor should look like and how they should behave. You will also form an opinion of what they will not look like and how you do not wish to be. Both of these value judgements will help you become the type of nurse you can emulate. This chapter, then, examines some of the features or expectations you might have of differing professional roles in order to help in your own development.

Expectations and the role of the student

What practitioners in health care can expect from students on professional courses in health has been a hotly debated issue among curriculum planners, practitioners and employers. In fact there are a variety of stakeholders who have strong views about what students should be able to do. The points, which need to be remembered, are that there are academic and professional standards and benchmarks associated with each course. These will influence and shape the role and expectations of students with whom you will come into contact. Students are allocated to a clinical placement in order to learn. Learning outcomes, aims and objectives will drive this learning. In a sense every student has a purpose for each placement. However, sometimes that purpose is neither clear nor shared by all parties involved. From a management viewpoint students' learning needs to be managed. The management of learning is dependent on the learning environment, the place where the learners interact with clients, patients and practitioners. There are a number of factors that managers of health care need to consider when planning learning and teaching for students. There is each student's stage that they are at in a particular course and programme. The student's abilities, attitudes, knowledge base and repertoire of skills should also be recognised as early in the placement as possible. There is also the context of care within a particular environment together with the quality of care delivered in such a context. All these will impinge on each student's learning.

There is often tension when you are a student rather than a member of staff because students may find it difficult to challenge practice. They may also find difficulty when they want to focus on an interesting point in practice while the rest of the team feel that they should be getting on with the tasks required of them.

The role of students is therefore dependent on a combination of elements, which need to be managed effectively if all parties involved are going to derive maximum benefit. It involves a partnership between the educational providers, practitioners, managers and, not least, the students themselves. However, from a placement perspective, learning can be structured or unstructured. Students will need support from mentors and in return they are expected to endorse the work ethics and be active and responsible for achieving specific learning outcomes or objectives for a given placement. An understanding of the student's role is therefore dependent on clear and effective communication among the student's educational providers, practitioners who support students in the field and managers who are responsible for organising and delivering health care.

- A student has been allocated to work with you for a period of four weeks.
- Identify the factors that must be considered in the planning of the student's learning and teaching in order to ensure realistic and unambiguous expectations for both the student and practitioners with whom they will be working.

Expectations of a newly qualified member of staff

One of the best-known definitions of the role of the nurse, and indeed this could be applied to all health care professionals, is that proposed by Virginia Henderson (1966) which states that:

> The unique function of the nurse is to assist the individual, sick or well, in the performance of those activities contributing to health or its recovery (or a peaceful death) that he would perform unaided if he had the strength, will or knowledge, and to do this in such a way as to help him gain independence as rapidly as possible.

This concept can be applied to any nursing branch but, as Henderson (1979) points out, it must also take into account the value systems of society at the time that the care is being delivered.

Whenever you take up a new post as a staff member, the expectation from your employer will relate to your ability to engage in and maintain a high standard of care. You will be expected to develop excellent communication skills, both verbal

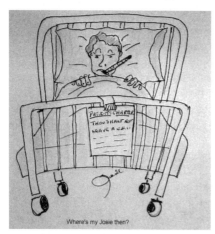

Where's my Josie then?

and written. In addition you will be expected to keep yourself up to date as well as being flexible in your approach to work. These expectations may sound a bit daunting at first; however, further analysis will reveal to you that by dint of having completed your education programme your competence in all of them will have been assessed. The areas in which your competence will have already been assessed in your professional course are care delivery, professional, managerial, education, administrative and general behaviour.

Care delivery

The expectations of your performance will be dependent on the philosophy and culture of the organisation and the particular type of health care activities that your course has prepared you for within that context. You will be expected to assess, plan, implement and evaluate care within the standards and philosophy of the organisation. Therefore it will be important for you to be familiar with those issues, policies, procedures and systems that are being operationalised in the workplace. There is an expectation that you will contribute to a high standard of care and develop effective relationships with clients/patients and relatives at all levels.

Professional

The term 'professional' is used in this context to convey the idea that health care workers who have a specific qualification that includes registration with a statutory body are expected to display behaviour that is consistent with a specific code. In this sense professional behaviour expected of you will include being courteous, non-judgemental, respectful and objective with patients and relatives at all times. In addition to your behaviour there is also an expectation that your knowledge base and practice will be supported by evidence derived from research and good practice.

Managerial

As part of your role you will be expected to be responsible for the care of a group of patients or clients. However, there will be support from senior colleagues initially. In that role your decision-making and problem-solving skills will be applied and tested. You will have to decide on priorities of care and the use of resources within your control and disposal. The organisation and management of the care of a group of clients/patients is going to be your direct responsibility. In that pursuit you will be expected to cope with some aspects of change as well as being able to delegate, monitor and supervise junior staff who are working in your team. You may also be invited to participate in clinical audit and other activities that involve collecting information and reviewing care.

Education

Health care professionals are expected to engage in educational activities within their sphere of work. This engagement covers a spectrum of activities that include direct involvement with clients/patients and relatives as well as colleagues or other members of personnel. This engagement is normally influenced by two major elements: first, the nature and scope of the post and the intrinsic demands for giving information and helping others to understand, apply and use information to promote and contribute towards health promotion and health education in the pursuit of physical, social and mental wellbeing; second, supporting and facilitating the learning and development of junior colleagues and students. The expectations so far as this aspect of your new role is concerned will also be dependent on your personal interests and enthusiasm for sharing information and knowledge. Initially you will be supported and encouraged in creating learning opportunities for yourself with a view that, as you gain more confidence and greater expertise, you will be able to use your own initiative to create learning environments that are conducive to learning and development.

Administrative

You must have heard the word 'paperwork' being used as you interact with health care professionals. This is seen as a chore – it is not a popular aspect of most jobs and does not generally generate any enthusiasm. However, this is an important aspect of most roles. Administrative skills are critical in ensuring efficient organisational systems and business in order to help achieve goals and provide the services that users need. Of course some bureaucratic requirements are ill-conceived and cumbersome and need review and change. These aspects of organisational life are always going to be present in one way or the other, hence the need for constant evaluation and reassessment of performance and effectiveness. The expectations from you are the ability and capacity to use the existing and current systems that are in place in the workplace. These may include ordering stocks and supplies that you will require, requesting leave and time off, communication with the multi-disciplinary/multi-agency teams and a variety of written communication activities which enable the smooth running of the workplace.

General

There are some expectations that all employers expect from their new recruits. Therefore they have been categorised as general. These include the following behaviours: punctuality, reliability, responsiblity, accountability and a show of enthusiasm for the post.

Managing for the first time

So the day has arrived when you are going to be in charge, alone for the first time. It is to be hoped that you will have been able to experience this aspect of your work, in a supported manner, during the latter few months of your education and training and through the preceptorship time immediately following qualification. Let us go back to the beginning, when you first entered your profession.

- What did you think a newly qualified nurse, midwife or health visitor did?
- What did you think their responsibilities were?
- How have your perceptions changed today?

Buckenham (1988) found that the perceptions of students changed during training in that first-year students thought more about the actual delivery of health care whereas third-year students thought that the clinical aspects of the job were less important than the effective management aspects. Whatever course you undertake, it appears that many qualified practitioners still feel unprepared for the management aspect of the role. In 1974 Kramer called this feeling the 'Reality Shock', when the feelings of dread, terror and fear abound. It is through exposure to management theory and supervised exposure to practice that nurses, midwives and health visitors are assisted in coming to terms with being in charge.

> What do you think you will do when you are first left in charge?

You may have thought of many things but whatever your list contains it will lead on to other questions, such as: will people be happy with me and will they do what I ask? Is my knowledge sufficient? Will I be able to cope? What will I be expected to cope with? All of these relate back to the art of delegation but also to the competencies for a first-level nurse stated in the now obsolete rules related to nursing. These have been superseded by those competencies set out in Education in Focus (English National Board for Nursing, Midwifery and Health Visiting 2000). Given the large number of different aspects of the job, the issues discussed within this book take on great importance. Lathlean and Corner (1991) found that half of the newly qualified nurses they looked at had taken total charge of their ward areas within the

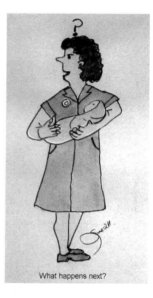

What happens next?

first month of qualification. Earlier Humphries (1987) found that almost a quarter of those studied 'were frequently left in charge despite the acute nature of the wards and (their own) inexperience'.

You may think that today professionals are being trained to manage without having sufficient experience with 'hands-on' care and that, rather than patients' or clients' needs and care coming first, the management role is more significant. Alternatively you might think that you would be managing the care of one patient or client rather than a group. Naturally if you are to be a midwife you will be caring for just one patient and her child during labour but within an ante- or post-natal ward it will be with a group.

Managing the ward must be separated from managing nursing work on an individual or team basis. Certainly you must be able to manage your time effectively if you are ever just to 'get through the day' delivering the best care possible to your patients/clients. It is vital to remember, at all times, that effective management skills are essential to effective patient care but the patients must come first. It might be useful, at this point, to list elements of the role of the nurse, midwife or health visitor as a manager. Table 4.1 attempts to examine a variety of roles encompassed and discussed within this book. With all these aspects and others, you might consider that it is little wonder that we sometimes think that registered nurses are people who 'nurse the nurses' station rather than the patient'.

Table 4.1 Role of the nurse, midwife or health visitor as a manager

Managing yourself	Managing the transition and coping with the 'reality shock' Effective time management Managing stress	
Managing the team within the Patient's Charter	Sharing administrative jobs Managing total patient care Clinical management Patients' rights Law and ethics	
Managing the clinical environment	Unit profile Physical environment Standards Nursing team Health and safety	Nurses' day Skill mix/off duty Patient/client day Resource control

Adapted from Lathlean et al (1987) Becoming a Staff Nurse

Accountability and the Code of Professional Conduct

Accountability means being held to ultimate account for a responsibility given to you. One simple definition may be 'The process by which responsibility is publicly addressed and reported on' (Hinchcliff 1999). Marquis and Huston (1998) give a broader moralistic view when they define accountability as 'Morally, internalising responsibility. It is an agreement to accept the consequences of actions'. This definition implies a personal thought process that is more than just an expectation of a job or a position.

In small health organisations like a 'single-handed' general practice, it may only be the doctor who is accountable for the service they provide. However, the health service is made up of many larger organisations where there are many people who manage others. The chief executive of a large health Trust is *accountable* for the total performance of their organisation.

Why do you think it is important to have this level of accountability in health care?

The health service is a specific area where patients may not know whether they are receiving good or bad care, particularly when they are very ill or disabled. The general public have now become very aware that they have particular rights and expectations from their health service. They are now demanding more accountability for public health services.

Nurses, midwives and health visitors in particular work in a very privileged position of trust and need to respect confidences and privacy and use their integrity when managing the care of individuals. The general public put a lot of trust and value in health care personnel when they come into contact with the health service and are often very vulnerable when they are in a highly dependent state. The concept of 'duty of care' is also important. Young (1995, p. 13) defines this term in the following way: 'a person must take reasonable care to avoid acts or omissions that he can reasonably foresee would be likely to injure a person directly affected by those acts'. Personal accountability as a nurse, midwife or health visitor is laid down within the requirements of the regulating and registering body of the UKCC. The UKCC (1992) in the *Code of Professional Conduct* identifies that each registered nurse, midwife or health visitor is personally accountable for their practice. Sixteen aspects of professional practice that accountability affects are identified and it is against these aspects that professional disciplinary and legal action may be judged. *The Code of Professional Conduct* highlights that registered practitioners are not only accountable to their line management but, importantly, to their individual patients and clients, society and also their profession. Interestingly, the Code highlights that personal accountability of practice may involve acts of omission or commission. This means that there may be aspects of care given that do not reach the standard expected that you may be held to account for and there may also be care aspects that have been neglected.

Nurse B is carrying out a medicine round in a ward at night. Mr C, who is in a very anxious state, is prescribed temazepam. Nurse B is unable to find the drug in the trolley. What should the nurse do?

- Identify some of the professional responsibilities she may face.
- What action should she take, remembering that she is accountable for acts of commission and omission?

She should take a reasonable period of time to try to locate the drug from another ward. If she has no staff to send to look for the drug, she could ask the nurse manager. If the drug was 'non-urgent' she may have to make a decision whether the drug could be safely omitted and given the next morning and whether it was important to contact the house officer. Can you think of some 'non-urgent' drugs? Some bowel preparations such as Lactulose may be considered to be non-urgent.

However, as the temazepam is important, the nurse should telephone the doctor if the drug cannot be found in the hospital. The doctor may wish to prescribe something else to ease the patient's anxiety.

- Imagine that the doctor feels there is little point writing up another drug and the temazepam can be safely omitted.
- Should the nurse inform the patient that she could not find his medication?

Employment accountability

Accountability is also set out under a contract of employment, so all employees will be accountable to their employing organisation. This is true even for the top person in an organisation like a chief executive. However, in order to be held accountable for managing large organisations it is fundamental that, for the top people to be effective, delegation will be necessary, right down the hierarchical line. Registered practitioners are accountable to their line manager for their own actions and the actions of their subordinates in getting the job done to the expected standard. Their subordinates, such as health care assistants, are responsible for doing the job required of them while on duty and will be contractually accountable to the registered practitioner. Students may also be held to account for their professional behaviour to both the university and the Trust educational confederation (which purchase the educational places).

The following roles in a clinical area demonstrate examples of accountability:

- Sister
  - accountability (ultimate ward responsibility)
  - seeing that the job gets done; standard of results achieved by subordinates
- Staff nurse
  - authority and responsibility
  - right to take action and make decisions
  - an obligation to perform the job with possible reprimand for unsatisfactory performance
- Health care assistant/student
  - authority and responsibility
  - right to take actions and make decisions
  - an obligation to perform the job with possible reprimand for unsatisfactory performance

Nurses, midwives and health visitors are accountable to:
- themselves
- their patients and clients
- society and the general public
- nursing midwifery and health visiting profession
- employers and line managers.

Of course this type of accountability is also true for all health care professionals.

It is useful at this point to distinguish between the terms 'delegation', 'authority' and 'responsibility'.

See if you can define the following terms:

Delegation means..................

Authority means.....................

Responsibility means...............

Did you find it difficult to put words to some of these concepts? You may have found it easier to define the action of delegation rather than the last two. Here are some suggestions of meanings.

- *Delegation* means the conferring of a special authority from a higher authority. It involves a two-part responsibility. The one to whom authority is delegated becomes responsible to the superior for doing the job, but the superior remains responsible for getting the job done.
- *Authority* is the right to take action or make decisions, which legitimises the exercise of power within an organisation.
- *Responsibility* involves an obligation to perform certain duties or make certain decisions and having to accept any reprimand from the manager for unsatisfactory performance.

Accountability to the public

Over the years, the general public's expectations of their National Health Service have been raised. Improved health technology, media coverage and the available use of the Internet has meant that the public have had more information on medical and caring advances. Indeed, at the beginning of the 1990s, the Conservative Government instigated a 'Charterism' ethos to their policies. There was a wave of charters for all public services, highlighting the public's rights and expectations.

The Patient's Charter

The Citizen's Charter led the way for the Patient's Charter (1992) which set out and distinguished between various expectations and rights for all patients. Its aim was to improve quality through national standards and focus on the needs of the 'consumer' of health services.

What do you think is the difference between a right and an expectation?

A *right* implies a legal or moral context whereas an *expectation* implies hope or desirability.

Do you know what some of the expectations are that are mentioned in the Patient's Charter?

The statements in Table 4.2 signal the type of service that the government hoped the NHS would deliver. However, you might detect that there is no legal duty for the NHS to meet the expectations given within these statements.

Table 4.2 Health service expectations (Patient's Charter 1992)

The expectations of the Patient's Charter are that:

- it will be easy to use
- children will be seen by specialists
- name badges, enquiry points, clear sign-posting and displayed local standards will be evident
- there will be respect for privacy, dignity, religious and cultural beliefs
- the Health Authority will send you a GP list or find you a GP in two working days; medical records will be sent on within six weeks (two days if urgent)
- you can expect to be informed about treatment times, readmission, standards and discharge decisions
- there will be notification of appointment times
- a bed will be ready as soon as possible, with single-sex washing and toilet facilities in a clean, safe environment
- a qualified nurse, midwife or health visitor will be responsible for your care
- a hospital food policy will be available in writing
- there will be community visit appointments and visiting standards
- there will be optometrist standards set with vision and dental charges
- there will be pharmacy standards set
- ambulance times will be set.

What do you know about the rights of patients?

Take a moment to think about these statements and identify which focus on rights?

Where does accountability for these rights rest?

The rights in the Charter, outlined in Table 4.3, focus on access to primary and secondary care with an emphasis on physical illness, medicine and treatment. Mental health, learning disability and maternity care have limited visibility. What does this say about rights to nursing, midwifery and health visiting care? How do these rights affect your particular branch of health care?

Table 4.5 Rights of patients (Patient's Charter 1992)

The Patient's Charter states that the rights of patients are:

1. To receive health care on the basis of your clinical need, not on your ability to pay, your lifestyle or any other factor.
2. To be registered with a GP and be able to change doctor easily and quickly.
3. To receive emergency care at any time through your GP, emergency ambulance service and hospital A/E departments.
4. To be offered a health check on joining a doctor's list for the first time.
5. To be offered a health check if you are between 16 and 74 years old and have not seen your GP in the last three years.
6. To be offered a health check once a year in the GP surgery or at home, if you are over 75 years old.
7. To receive information about your GP services and see a copy of your practice leaflet on request.
8. To be referred to a consultant acceptable to you when your GP thinks it necessary and to be referred for a second opinion if you and the GP agree that this is desirable.
9. To have appropriate drugs and medicines prescribed and decide which pharmacy you wish to use.
10. To be given a clear explanation of any treatment proposed, including any risks and any alternatives, before you decide whether you agree to the treatment.
11. To have access to health records, subject to any limitations in the law and to know that those working for the NHS are under a legal duty to keep their contents confidential.
12. To choose whether or not you wish to take part in medical research or medical student training.
13. To be given detailed information on local health services, including quality standards and maximum waiting times.
14. To be told before you go into hospital whether it is planned to care for you in a ward for men and women.

15. To be guaranteed admission for treatment by a specific date no later than two years from the date that the consultant places you on the waiting list.

16. That if you are registered with a dentist, to receive advice in an emergency and treatmenty if your dentist considers it necessary.

17. That after a vision test, you will receive a signed written prescription to receive glasses and be able to take this to any optometrist or dispensing optician of your choice. If you do not need glasses, to have a written statement telling you this.

18. To have any complaints about the NHS services – whoever provides them – investigated and to receive a full and prompt written reply from the chief executive or general manager.

There are some obvious areas where nursing, midwifery and health visiting are accountable within the context of these rights, such as:

- in provision of health care based on clinical need
- in provision of emergency care
- allowing access to health records
- referring patients to doctors when appropriate drugs and medications are required
- maintaining confidentiality.

The Patient's Charter could be described as a politically motivated document, which highlights a move away from paternalism towards patient autonomy, or even as a response to the values of consumerism within society. This may have the outcome of pacifying the electorate. However, the Patient's Charter uses statements that are not always clear in law but are more symbolic. It is interesting to see how much commitment there has been to these statements over the past few years and what limitations have been experienced in meeting these rights. For instance, there is no right to have dentistry services on the NHS and no standard of the type of dentistry service that needs to be provided by those existing NHS dentists for routine care. Interestingly, registration with an NHS dentist now only lasts for *fifteen months* and re-registration will require at least an annual dental check. This means that the NHS has effectively reduced the service.

On the other hand, the Charter did give nurses and midwives an opportunity to become more involved with care management issues and to keep pace with the expectations of patients and clients through involvement in audits and project work.

Legal and ethical issues

Accountability within the health service is influenced by employment, criminal, civil and professional action. Legal and ethical issues are therefore important professional considerations. Ethics is the study of what our conduct and actions *ought to be* (rather than what it actually is) with respect to others, the environment and ourselves. It is sometimes difficult to separate out ethics and legal issues.

It is interesting to note that health care professionals, once held in high esteem, are now less trusted and are held to account more than before as cases where individuals who have abused their autonomy for personal satisfaction and criminal activities have become more visible. The health care industry is also facing the ethical problem of trying to meet infinite demand with finite resources. Financial, physical and human resources are being allocated on a priority basis. This has always been the case but there is more transparency than before. The implications of these points are that ethical considerations form an important component of health care management. Ethical dilemmas also face clinical staff daily. Haddad (1992) defines an ethical dilemma as a novel, complex and ambiguous problem that does not lend itself to programmed or routine problem solving for which a precedent has been set. In other words, ethical dilemmas are forms of 'messy' problems.

> Can you make a note of any recent clinical problems where you felt that ethics played a part?

It may be that you have thought about resuscitation decisions made in your area or perhaps decisions about withholding medical treatment for certain groups of people such as the elderly, those with a disability or those who have problems considered self-inflicted. You may have identified that screening for certain abnormalities may also pose ethical decisions. The use of *ethical principles* is useful in examining the issues within any ethical dilemma. Marquis and Huston (1998) identify the following:

- *Autonomy*: This infers freedom of choice or accepting the responsibility for one's choice. Legal items around the right to self-determination support this moral principle.
- *Beneficence*: This refers to the point that actions and decisions should be taken in order to promote good. Non-maleficence goes further: if one cannot do good, then at least one should do no harm.
- *Paternalism*: This principle is related to the positive good that could occur when one individual makes decisions on behalf of another individual. This has to be balanced with the issue where paternalism may limit freedom of choice for another. Paternalism is possibly only justified to prevent harm to others.
- *Utility*: This principle reflects a belief in utilitarianism, where common good outweighs what is good for an individual. This justifies paternalism in also restricting the choice of the individual.
- *Justice*: This principle is based on the point that equals should be treated equally and 'unequals' should be treated according to their diversity.
- *Truth telling and deception*: This refers to the extent to which an individual will go to tell the truth or accept deception.

To be a good ethical problem solver, you must become more self-aware about your own values and beliefs concerning rights, duties and goals of individuals.

Legal issues

These issues stem from the statutes and the law of the land. As a health care professional, you should be aware of the legal controls surrounding your practice.

Professional negligence in health care involves any form of malpractice. Malpractice is the failure of a professional with a body of knowledge to act in what is considered a reasonable and prudent manner. This would imply a manner expected of the average health care professional in that discipline, based on expected judgements, foresight, intelligence and skill. Health care professionals hold their own personal liability concerning practice. Fletcher and Buka (1999, p. 53) identify that it is a professional code of conduct that will enable a judge to decide whether a practitioner was acting within the expectations of their particular profession. This point is known as the Bolam Test from a notable legal test case (*Bolam v. Friern Hospital Management Committee* (1957) 1 WLR 582; (1957) All ER 118). Issues such as the position of trust afforded to the professional and the action taken to protect patients' or clients' best interests will be of particular interest in the eyes of the law.

Employers have no legal right within a contract of employment to ask you to account for your professional action. They could however, bring a disciplinary case against you if you failed to account for care, which was deemed poor, and this could thus lead to redundancy. It is only when there is a legal inquiry (criminal or civil) that a professional may need to go to a Court of Law, e.g. in child protection, murder or assault/harm cases, and that a health professional may have to account for their action. In legal inquires, the health profession may have to account for any breach in their 'duty to care'.

The Council of Nursing and Midwifery (replacing the UKCC/ENB 2001) may also ask professionals to account for their actions but they have no statutory right to force an account. They can, however, through their disciplinary procedures make certain decisions concerning registration. Whether through employment, the law or the Council of Nursing and Midwifery, withholding evidence or an account of practice may ultimately jeopardise your job prospects, your citizenship and/or your professional registration.

It is important therefore that all health care professionals keep up to date with legislation and the implications of the Code of Professional Conduct (UKCC 1992).

Accountability and quality

Accountability for practice involves moving with the times and not just relying on what was taught during initial training. Knowledge and skills of yesteryear will not be adequate to meet the demands of today and the future.

Therefore professional responsibility involves being accountable for updating these areas and being research minded. It is about a personal philosophy of *continuous improvement*.

How do you see yourself addressing this issue in your professional career?

It means that you have to be keen to keep on learning for the rest of your working life in order to improve your practice. This may be a tall order for some individuals! The government acknowledges the need for *life-long learning* which is a thread running through the document *A First Class Service* (Department of Health 1999). This health policy aims to address the NHS — from a consumer focus in the direction of *professional accountability* in the public domain. How health professionals account for and accept their role in delivering quality services is now underpinned in the concepts of *clinical governance* and *shared governance*. The Department of Health (1999, p. 33) defines clinical governance as:

> a framework through which NHS organisations are accountable for continuously improving the quality of their services and safeguarding high standards of care by creating an environment in which excellence in clinical care can flourish.

Although this will be covered in Chapter 11, it is useful to see here that the government is making an attempt to include and monitor the professional's perception of quality health care.

Why do you think this is important?

Chapter 11 may help you here. Governance concerns the style of management and leadership in an organisation and involves taking on board responsibility, regulation and control within health care. Some health professionals will fear accountability and responsibility and will require support through the organisation and through professional bodies. However, Castledine (1999) highlights that although some nurses do not want any more professional authority and accountability. Clinical governance could be the link between the individual nurse showing autonomy and accountability, and, linking with others, could demonstrate a collective interest in quality practice that can be delivered to the organisation.

Reflection and reflective practice

You may think that reflection has very little to do with you as a student but, whether you examine your private life or your professional one, there are times when you will think 'that didn't go too well' or 'that was brilliant'. Reflection is looking at what factors made something go well or, conversely, go badly (particularly when linking theory to practice) and learning from this. Evaluation and critical thinking skills can then develop. A definition offered by the American Unitarian Association (1883) cited by Funk (1946) stated:

> Reflection – The act or habit of directing the mind thoughtfully and attentively to something that has previously occupied it; continued consideration or meditation, or the result of it; thought; as, reflection increases wisdom.

> The learning commonly gathered from books is of less worth than the truths we gain from experience and reflection. (Changing Works, Laboring Classes, p. 51, AUA (1883))

The overall experience of reflection may be humbling, disturbing, boring or even inspirational but, whatever it is, it will be a learning experience. Street (1991) asserts that reflection in nursing is seen as a way to:

> Empower nurses to become fully cognisant of their own knowledge and actions, the personal and professional histories which have shaped them, the symbols and images inherent in the language they use, the myths and metaphors which sustain them in practice, their nursing experiences, and the potentialities and constraints of their work setting. (Street 1991)

It is, however, difficult to achieve. In the beginning there is usually a tendency to be descriptive rather than analytical (but do not worry about this for as you progress through your educational programme your reflections will become more analytical as you have more experiences to draw upon). Reflective practice in nursing is based on the works of people like Schön (1991, 1987), Kolb (1984), Benner (1984), Boud, et al. (1985), Gibbs (1988) and Johns (1998).

Schön (1991) describes a crisis of confidence in the professions, witnessed by well-publicised scandals in which highly esteemed individuals have misused their autonomy. In order to allay the fears of the general public and to uphold the professional status to which we aspire, we must be seen to be able to justify our actions, develop professional knowledge and uphold standards. John Kennedy (1962), cited in Schön (1991), urged young people to 'participate ... in the solution of the problems that pour upon us, requiring the most sophisticated solution to complex and obstinate issues.' Being responsible for our actions is vital but in order to be responsible we must understand what we are doing; it is here that reflection comes into its own. Wilkinson (1999) suggests that you should keep a reflective diary in order to record your experiences during any placement, and later when you are qualified this practice would be maintained for your portfolio. This does not mean that you should be writing 'Dear diary' every day, but when you learn something new or when you look back and think about an area of your work. Within this diary you might record reflections before action (considering what the desired outcome is), in action (during the practice event) and on action (following the practice event). Whatever the stage of your reflection, you should record your thoughts as soon as practicably possible, remembering to conform to the UKCC Code of Professional Conduct in relation to confidentiality. Confidentiality relates not only to the patient but also to the Trust, to colleagues and to the environment in which you are working. The important element is to learn from your experience.

How do you see yourself addressing this issue in your professional career?

Differing theorists offer a variety of ways but in order for the process to have meaning for you it is often useful to set yourself a series of questions which can be addressed in turn.

- *What happened or what was going to happen?*
  - Include the context of the experience and why it was important to you.
- *What were your feelings and thoughts?*
  - What were you thinking and feeling before, during and after the event?
  - What were others thinking and feeling?
  - What did you find most demanding about the experience?
- *What was good and what was bad about the overall experience?*
  - What was successful/what could be improved?
  - What influenced your decision making?
- *What sense can you make of this experience?*
  - What have you learnt and what are the important issues for patient/client care?
- *What else could have been done?*
  - What other choices of action did you have?
  - What might have been the outcome of these choices?
- *Action plan*
  - How will all this influence your further practice?
  - What else do you now need to do/learn?

It is useful to follow this format when reflecting on action. By answering the questions posed you will learn from experience and be able to justify your actions in the future. Together with this you will be fulfilling the need to maintain a portfolio demonstrating learning and updating of practice. As part of the Clinical Governance initiative (Chapter 11), all health care professionals will be required to undertake professional development continuously. Mandatory updating is required by the new Nursing and Midwifery Council. A portfolio of evidence is therefore very useful. As a student you will be learning or trying to remember vast quantities of information; by writing things down we remember them more easily. Much more could be written about this area of practice but we would direct you to the References and Further reading sections on p. 73–4 to enhance your reflective practice.

Conclusion

Within this chapter we have examined a variety of issues related to the way we perceive ourselves, and the ways others might see us. The benefits of really trying to identify our own strengths and weaknesses together with their associated opportunities and threats lead us to decide what our ideal role model is and the ways of reaching that goal. In order to do this, we first examined the expectations and role of the student nurse, midwife or health visitor before going on to look at the expectations of the newly qualified member of staff. Managing for the first time is stressful, but we can more easily come to terms with the demands of being in charge of a clinical area/group of patients/clients through reflection before the event (i.e. reflection before action).

It has been shown that all these actions and thoughts must relate to the Code of Professional Conduct and we are governed by this Code. The effects of this, together with the Patient's Charter, were debated and linked to patient/client care.

Summary of key points

This chapter has examined the following areas:

- **Expectations and role of the student:** Looking at the benefit of learning outcomes and placements in order to give breadth of experience to build upon.

- **Expectations of a newly qualified member of staff:** Examined six aspects of the role in terms of care delivery, professional, managerial, education, administrative and general behaviour, demonstrating how these areas impact on the role.

- **Managing for the first time:** Started by looking at initial thoughts of the role on entry to the educational programme and how they might have changed during the programme.

- **Accountability and the Code of Professional Conduct:** Accountability was defined and its impact on work practices discussed. Within this a variety of scenarios were examined: employment accountability; accountability to the public; the Patient's Charter; legal and ethical issues; accountability and quality.

- **Reflection and reflective practice:** Was briefly examined, recognising that the subject area was vast. Suggestions were made to assist students in developing their roles and portfolios by becoming reflective practitioners.

References

Benner P (1984) *From Novice to Expert.* Addison-Wesley

Boud D, Keogh R and Walker D (1985) *Reflection: Turning Experience into Learning,* Kogan Page

Buckenham M A (1988) Student nurse perception of the staff nurse role, *Journal of Advanced Nursing,* **13**, 662–70

Castledine G (1999) *Writing, Documentation and Communication Skills for Nurses,* Quay

Department of Health (1992) *The Patient's Charter,* HMSO

Department of Health (1999) *A First Class Service,* HMSO

English National Board for Nursing, Midwifery and Health Visiting (2000) *Education in Focus – Strengthening Pre-Registration Nursing and Midwifery Education (Curriculum Guidance and Requirements),* ENB

Fletcher L and Buka P (1999) *A Legal Framework for Caring,* Macmillan

Funk I K (ed.) (1946) *New Standard Dictionary of the English Language,* Funk & Wagnalls

Gibbs G (1988) *Learning by Doing: Developing Teaching Skills,* Further Education Unit, Oxford Polytechnic

Haddad A M (1992) Ethical problems in health care, *Journal of Advanced Nursing* **22** (3), 46–51

Henderson V (1966) *The Nature of Nursing,* Collier-Macmillan

Henderson V (1979) Preserving the essence of nursing in a technological age, *Nursing Times* **75** (47), 2012–13

Hinchliff S (1999) *The Practitioner as a Teacher* (2nd edn) Baillière Tindall/RCN

Humphries A (1987) The transition from student to staff nurse. Unpublished BSc Thesis, Leicester University. Cited in Lathlean and Corner (1991)

Johns C, (1996) Visualising and realising caring in practice through guided reflection, *Journal of Advanced Nursing* **24**, 1135–73

Kolb D A (1984) *Experiential Learning: Experience as the Source of Learning and Development,* Prentice Hall.

Kramer M (1974) *Reality Shock – Why Nurses Leave Nursing,* Mosby

Lathlean J and Corner J (1991) (eds) *Becoming a Staff Nurse – A Guide to the Role of the Newly Registered Nurse,* Prentice Hall

Marquis B L and Huston C J (1998) *Leadership Roles and Management Functions in Nursing* (3rd edn) Lippincott

Schön D A (1987) *Educating the Reflective Practitioner: Toward a New Design for Teaching and Learning in the Professions,* Jossey-Bass

Schön D A (1991) *The Reflective Practitioner: How Professionals Think in Action*, Basic Books

Street A (1991) From image to action-reflection in nursing practice, Deakin University, Geelong. Cited in Palmer A, Burns S and Bulman C (eds) (1994) *Reflective Practice in Nursing: The Growth of the Reflective Practitioner*, Blackwell Science.

UKCC (1992) *Code of Professional Conduct*, UKCC

Wilkinson J (1999) Implementing reflective practice, *Nursing Standard*, **13** (21), 36–40

Young A (1995) The legal dimension, in Tingle J and Cribb A (eds) *Nursing Law and Ethics*, Blackwell Scientific

Further reading

Brubacher J W, Case C W and Reagan T G (1994) *Becoming a Reflective Educator: How to Build a Culture of Inquiry in the Schools*, Corwin Press.

Burnard P (1988) The journal as an assessment and evaluation tool in nursing education, *Nurse Education Today*, **8**, 105–7

Johns C, Freshwater D (eds) (1998) *Transforming Nursing through Reflective Practice*, Blackwell Science

Johns C (1995) Framing learning through reflection, *Journal of Advanced Nursing*, **22**, 226–34

Palmer A, Burns S and Bulman C (1994) *Reflective Practice in Nursing – The Growth of the Professional Practitioner*, Blackwell Science.

Rudduck J (1991) *Innovation and Change*, Open University Press

Vroom V (1964) *Work & Motivation*, Wiley

Yelloly M and Henkel M (eds) (1995) *Learning and Teaching in Social Work: Towards Reflective Practice*, Jessica Kingsley

Part

II

The team

5

Organising care

By the end of this chapter you will have had the opportunity to:

- recognise the various methods of organising the nursing structure to deliver quality care
- recognise the cultural and structural values concerning the concept of Nursing Development Units
- discuss the advantages and disadvantages of various nursing structures on patient care

Introduction

The way that nurses organise their work activities so that organisational and patient goals are met have been the focus of improving care in the last twenty to thirty years. Various care delivery methods have been researched in terms of their effectiveness and efficiency. This chapter deals with the structure of care delivery, as it evolved historically in nursing, and aims to explore the link between the structure and effectiveness of patient care delivery. Table 5.1 demonstrates the order in which developments will be discussed throughout the chapter.

Table 5.1 Developing nursing management and philosophies of care – sequence of UK events

	Nursing management	Philosophy of care
1940s–1960s	Task allocation	
1950s	Team nursing	Holistic care
1960s	Patient allocation	The nursing process
Early 1980s	Team nursing	Nursing models
1981	Nursing Development Units	Individualised care
Late 1980s	Primary nursing	Individualised care
1991	Care programme approach	Multi-disciplinary approach

Task allocation

Task allocation may be thought of as being one of the most efficient ways of delivering nursing care as it 'gets the job done'. Tasks were allocated according to seniority so that junior nurses dealt with 'essential care' while the senior nurses addressed the complex management tasks (Figure 5.1).

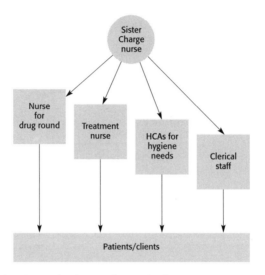

Figure 5.1 Functional or task-orientated organization

The shortage of nurses during the 1940s and 1950s demanded a realistic and down-to-earth approach to nursing. Traditional nursing in hospitals (and also in the community) was organised in such a way that it was sometimes fragmented and broken down into small tasks. This task-orientated climate, linked to the management of the disease process, was not universal but was seen as a security blanket for students and staff, because of the heavy reliance on an ever-changing student workforce as they moved on every three months. Evidence includes the use of 'workbooks', which highlighted who would 'do the observations, bedpans' etc.; the 'back book'; the bath book; and many other forms of documenting tasks and their completion (Table 5.2).

Indeed, student nurses of the 1960s learned to deliver care in this way. Duberley (1977) argued strongly that

> carrying out both medical orders and routine are highly valued, and that British nursing generally offers a service based largely on medical diagnosis, the consultant's ward round and/or the ward sister's preference.

Table 5.2 Sample page from a workbook, 1 September 1964

Morning:		
M A Tress	1st year student	Bed baths; backs
P Key	1st year student	Bedpans; lockers
W Ounds	2nd year student	Dressings; observations
I C Kerr	3rd year student	Drugs; observations
A S Prinn	Staff Nurse	Drugs; dressings
A Tinkle	Nursing Auxiliary	Bed baths; bedpans; flowers
E McCafferty	Sister	Ward round
Afternoon:		
J Samuels	1st year student	Bed baths; backs
P Wright	1st year student	Bedpans; hair washing
W Jones	2nd year student	Hair washing
A Long	3rd year student	Drugs; observations
S Grey	Staff Nurse	Drugs
M John	Nursing Auxiliary	Bedpans; flowers
E McCafferty	Sister	Ward round

It fits in well with the notion of control within a hierarchical organisation like the National Health Service and in particular with the need for the person in charge to exhibit total control of their sphere of authority.

- Examine a clinical area or placement where you have been involved in this type of delivery of care.
- Can you list some of the advantages and disadvantages?

Advantages relate to the fact that the work gets done and the ward manager knows who is responsible for what and therefore who to 'blame' when work is not completed. Care tasks and simple practical skills can be learned quickly by junior or unqualified staff, leaving the qualified nurse free to respond to the doctors' prescriptions. Similarly, the pride experienced in completing a task when taking on that responsibility and the feeling of worth and a job well done are not to be ignored. On the other hand, the patient sees many different nurses and the nurses may become specialised in only one area, so leading to fragmented care; this reflected the level of knowledge at the time. Within many sectors of nursing, midwifery or health visiting task allocation is still used, for example within a clinic situation where repetitive tasks need to be done, e.g. measuring and weighing. However, Pearson and Vaughan (1986) highlighted the fact that this mode of delivery of care failed to consider the whole person and ignored other aspects, e.g. psychological, social and spiritual needs. This type of care delivery prevailed from the inception of the NHS in 1948 through to the late 1960s and early 1970s when the organisation of the NHS underwent a series of reviews. The improvement was thought to be in the form of 'patient allocation', which will be discussed later as it was sandwiched between the initial introduction of 'team nursing' in the 1950s and its re-emergence during the 1980s.

Team nursing

> Team Nursing enables continuity in allocation of nurses to work with patient groups while at the same time facilitating supervision of student nurses. (Clark and Copcutt 1997)

During the 1950s the concept of 'team nursing' was highlighted in the literature as an attempt to reduce problems associated with the functional organisation of patient care, i.e. task allocation, and focused on the patient, whose total needs were considered. Today the team has a range of grades and skills and within a clinical area there will be more than one team which addresses the individual care plans of its patients (Figure 5.2).

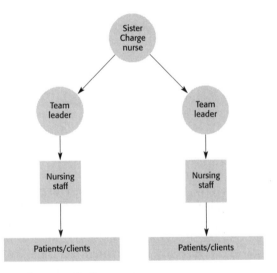

Figure 5.2 Team nursing organization

The terms 'patient-centred' and 'individualised' care were popularised in the 1960s to describe a new approach to health care delivery. This one-to-one therapeutic relationship is seen in many areas today including community, mental health and midwifery care. Indeed, if one examines the work of the midwife one can see that the delivery of care does not really fit into a 'team nursing' concept, except in ante- or post-natal wards. However, in the light of present-day changes in childbirth, efforts have been made to introduce the concept of mid-wifery teams in the community. The woman will know the specific group of midwives, whom she will have met during the ante-natal period. The members of this team will be at the same grade, as opposed to a team with a more broadly defined skill mix. Midwifery teams focus on the delivery event and this method of organisation achieves 24-hour cover.

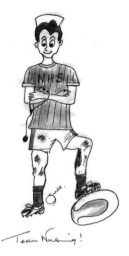

Team Nursing!

- Think about a situation you have been in where team nursing was effective.
- Why was it effective?
- Could it be effective for all disciplines of care delivery?
- In which areas do you think this type of care delivery may be of limited use?

Again, you may have highlighted that the team leader assesses the conditions and needs of all the patients and it is the team leader who assists team members in the delivery of care. Similarly, the team leader should coordinate patient activities and will attempt to use a democratic leadership style wherein the members are given autonomy and are able to contribute their own specialist skills or interests to the care needed. Most importantly, the patient knows the team and is able to build up a trusting relationship with them.

The disadvantages usually relate to poor communication and leadership styles. There may be insufficient time allowed for team care planning and communication; there may be inappropriate task allocation; and information may often flow in a 'top-down' direction with little or no 'bottom-up' flow. There may be blurred lines of responsibility, which may lead to errors/omissions and it is said that the care may still be fragmented in nature in the same way as for task allocation. Katherine Vestal (1987) argues that team nursing 'does not provide for continuity of care between care given or between shifts because assignments can change daily and patients are still confronted with single function people entering their room' (Vestal 1987). However, within a midwifery situation, particularly during labour, skill mix teams may well be inappropriate as the emphasis of care relies on the one-to-one relationships to gain cooperation and trust during delivery.

There has been a tremendous interest in primary care teams in the last decade. Recent literature points to the need for effective teamwork from all agencies (Audit Commission 1992, Department of Health 1993, Department of Health 1996). Case/care management is an example and is considered later. However, another view of teamwork in primary care is the integrated nursing team (Figure 5.3). This has been defined as:

a team of community based nurses from different disciplines working together within a primary care setting, pooling their skills, knowledge and ability in order to provide the most effective care for patients within a practice and the community it covers. (Health Visitors Association 1996)

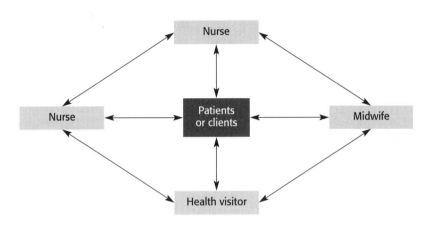

Figure 5.3 Integrated team

The internal 'nursing' team of general practice may include practice, psychiatric and district nurses, midwives and health visitors. This integrated teamwork on problem-solving projects often brings out innovative ideas, comradeship with members and satisfying outcomes for patients, staff and managers. They are action-centred and may lack bureaucratic processes that impede the task at hand; however, they do rely on good inter-relationships based on trust and respect.

Patient allocation

Here, rather than being directed towards a series of tasks, a nurse would be given a group of patients and was expected to care for their total needs. Running alongside the organisational changes of the 1970s came the expansion of the knowledge base relating to the need for psychological and social care, which in turn led to the recognition that task-dominated, physically orientated systems of delivery of care did not meet the needs of patients and clients. The term 'patient allocation' is now widely used and accepted and was interpreted as leading to the notion of 'holism' and 'holistic care'. In the early 1970s it was quite revolutionary and represented a major breakthrough from the hierarchical, accepted way of delivering care. Unfortunately, the nurse training of the day still focused on the 'medical model' so that the overall delivery of care did not change to any great degree and remained with the management of the disease process. It can be seen, then, that this did not appear to alter the overall philosophy of ward management. Liaison with other members of the multi-disciplinary team remained in the ward sister's domain. Alongside this 'the nursing process' was being implemented.

The nursing process

The nursing process offered a framework in which to construct a total package of care for an individual during their interaction with the health care teams. It focused on four areas: assessment, planning, implementation and evaluation. However, the introduction of this process was not well managed (Department of Health 1987) as the end users, the nurses, were not given the necessary knowledge base from which to work. The resulting problem was that the 'nursing process' (describing care) became confused with the system of organising the delivery of care (patient allocation) so that neither was effective and the concept of the nursing process became synonymous with additional and excessive paperwork. Medical staff and other professions allied to medicine saw this in a negative manner and felt that there was emphasis on paperwork at the expense of care delivery (Mitchell 1984).

Table 5.1 shows that there are many overlaps in the times that various strategies were employed and during the 1980s it was recognised that a model to support the nursing process was required. In the USA a variety of nurses had put forward models, e.g. Peplau (1952), Roy (1976), Orem (1980), Neuman (1982) and from England the best known is Roper *et al.* (1981). Texts related to these models are readily available. However, it would appear that in many care settings, where models are used, there will be a selection of a preferred model which will be used irrespective of patient needs, e.g. a patient who has a terminal illness could benefit from the use of Peplau's model rather than Orem's or Roper *et al.*'s model.

Primary nursing

The primary nursing approach means that an individual nurse takes responsibility for an individual patient throughout a period of treatment or hospital stay. It is believed that the USA may have used primary nursing in hospitals in the 1960s but it is likely that it was evolving at different rates across the world.

The primary nurse is responsible for planning and administrating care, including referrals to other agencies and discharge planning, for the period of time that the patient is in hospital or 'on the books' in the community. It is regarded as going further than the patient allocation model which was used from the 1960s (Figure 5.4). The role of the sister/charge nurse is now, in relation to the patient, more of an administrative and supportive nature for the primary nurse, unless, the sister/charge nurse is a primary nurse in their own right.

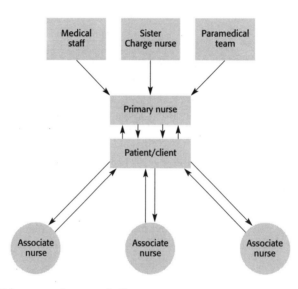

Figure 5.4 Primary nursing organization

Primary nursing allows a close therapeutic relationship between nurse and patient to develop, the patient and family know who is responsible and accountable for the care period and the primary nurse can also work in a professional and autonomous way, becoming accountable for the total care package. It also gives nurses a lot of job satisfaction. Community nursing had always used the primary nursing approach but was sometimes used alongside a task focus, i.e. district nurse visiting a home for the sole purpose of doing a dressing, giving eye drops, taking out sutures.

- Why do you think primary nursing works in the community?
- What are the problems associated with primary nursing in the acute sector?

You may have thought about the obvious problems of requiring care from several nurses during a 24-hour period in hospital, whereas in the community it is families, in the main, that care for the patients with the support of the nursing service. You might also have asked how the primary nurse could be totally responsible when there may be many dependency changes, and planning is required to meet those needs in hospital. In terms of treating patients as individuals with unique experiences that are dynamic during the day and night, the primary nurse is then expected to plan using a team approach. A patient may be assessed on admission by the primary nurse, be taken down to theatre by another nurse and be brought back from theatre by yet another nurse. There are plans that can be made in advance but what happens in an emergency or when theatre is delayed or cancelled? The primary nurse cannot be available at all times. Table 5.3 demonstrates how the primary nurse may hand over care to the associate nurse, a back-up for the primary nurse and who continues the care when the primary nurse is off duty or sick. The reality of ward 'off duty' being organised around primary and associate nurses creates extra problems for the person doing the 'off duty', especially in the light of the numbers of unqualified to qualified nurses. It also has implications for lack of staff development for evening and night staff in some wards.

Table 5.3 Primary nurse case study

Mr Singh is admitted to hospital with abdominal pains. The doctors suspect an acute obstructive condition which will require surgery. The patient and his family are apprehensive, not knowing what treatment he will be given, how long he will be off work, what he will be fed and how he will be cared for.

- The primary nurse comes in to the admission room smiling and introduces herself as Manjit: 'I am Manjit and I am your primary nurse.'
- She discusses the problems and the fears, asking Mr Singh about the pain, in Mr Singh's terms.
- She asks about his family, work, diet, sleep and coping mechanisms.
- She then tells them about the doctor's plan, encouraging them to ask questions, and says that she hopes to look after Mr Singh nearly as well as he would be at home.
- She asks Mr Singh's wife about travelling to see him and openly encourages her to be with her husband as much as possible. They identify members of the extended family who might help with the children and the travelling.
- Manjit shows the family the facilities in the room and the ward and allows the family to settle in.
- The doctor comes along and puts an IV in place and Manjit is there for Mr Singh. As she gives him some pain relief, Manjit discusses a care plan, which is later written out, stating the realistic goals and the ways Mr Singh will get back to independence.
- When she is going off duty that afternoon, Manjit lets Mr Singh know that she is going and introduces him to Paul, the associate nurse, who will be looking after him in her absence and taking him down to theatre.
- Manjit has already planned for Mr Singh's peri-operative, post-operative and discharge and knows she will be working with the hospital doctor, the community GP and the district nurses for the benefit of Mr Singh's recovery.

Ersser and Turton (1991) have evaluated primary nursing and question whether individualised care equates with patient satisfaction. They suggest that quality may be about nursing care but may also be about clean sheets, good food or a quiet environment. Primary nursing care does not always equate with competent practice but more proficient nurses may migrate to primary nursing environments for better job satisfaction.

Effective and efficient methods of care delivery will be affected by the patient dependency, the competencies of the staff on duty and the extra workload, e.g. ward rounds, ward clinics. Chapter 4 also highlighted roles and expectancy theory in relation to effort, and performance and positive outcomes for patient care. The way that a clinical area is organised does not always utilise one method or another: some areas organise their day staff into team nursing, with primary nursing occurring at night.

Named nurse, midwife or health visitor

Since the early 1990s acute units have become managed through the notion of directorates, whereby there is a medical manager, a nursing manager and a business manager identified. Within this system, nurses and midwives are professionally accountable but also managerially accountable to other members of the health care team. For a profession steeped in traditional accountability there have been major changes leading to broader managerial expectations (budget holding became the remit of some nursing and mid-

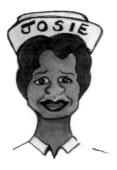

wifery managers). Together with this, clinical managers had to develop quality standards measured through the use of audit. Some standards related to those introduced within the Patient's Charter. The Patient's Charter (Department of Health 1992) led to the mandatory introduction of the named nurse as Charter Standard No. 8 states that 'A named nurse, midwife or health visitor will be responsible for your nursing or midwifery care.'

Dargan (1992) suggests that for named nursing to succeed, it should be seen as separate and distinct from primary nursing while accepting that its origins are within the primary nursing model. Wright (1997, cited in Dargan 1997) suggested that, with the emergence of various Patient's Charters, nurses were moved along a continuum from apathy to enthusiasm. Within the acute sector of care delivery the notion of developing the role of the named nurse was problematical.

- Are you putting the named nurse, midwife or health visitor into practice?
- How is this demonstrated/seen?
- Is it successful?

You might believe that you are putting it into practice – in some instances it may be so but within the acute setting it may only be in the form of 'lip service'. The name of the nurse may well be posted at the head of the bed, together with that of the consultant in charge of the case, but if you were to ask the patient to point out their named nurse, would they be able to do it? It is suggested that in many instances the patient would have to be prompted.

Tingle (1993) discusses three areas where a nurse may refuse to be a named nurse and not contravene the UKCC (1992) *Code of Professional Conduct*:

1. Nurse feels they are not ready to be a named nurse – the ward manager must be told and will then become legally liable for any negligent act performed by the nurse.
2. Nurse feels competent in most situations but not able to plan the nursing care for this particular patient.
3. Delegation of named nurses not correctly practised – i.e. the nurse is allocated to a patient in their absence, or just prior to annual leave or days off. However, if it is a long-stay unit this may not present a problem or valid reason.

So who can this named nurse, midwife or health visitor be?

You will probably come up with the answer that they must be a first-level practitioner. Good. But more important than that, they *must be there* for the majority of the time that the patient is in their care. You can see from this statement alone that meeting this basic requirement is perhaps one of the most difficult areas to address.

Table 5.4 offers a fourteen-point list of things the named nurse should be doing if this system is to be successful. Indeed, Florence Nightingale (1859 cited in van der Peet 1995) stated that 'it is better to know a patient in a certain condition than the condition from which the patient may suffer', thus putting the emphasis on the need for nursing rather than medical models.

Table 5.4 What should a Named Nurse do?

1. **Be aware** of their limits of freedom of choice in accepting patients.
2. **Conduct** their first meeting with their patient within 24 hours of admission.
3. **The meeting may be** with the patient, relatives/carer or both together.
4. **It would be ideal** if they were the patient's first point of contact on admission to the unit.
5. **After the first meeting** they must either:
   - accept the nursing care plan and update as necessary
   - amend the nursing care plan
   - write the appropriate nursing care plan
   - communicate any changes in nursing plans to the patient.
6. **Sign and date** their authorisation of the patient's nursing care plan.
7. **They must be able to** support the nursing care plan with relevant, continually updated practice-based research recommendations.
8. **Set and record** realistic measurable goals and target dates which are, if possible, mutually agreed between patients and themselves.
9. **Coordinate** the patient's care – within the accepted limits of multi-disciplinary support practices within the area.
10. **State** on the plan the prerequisites for discharge.
11. **Participate** in the nursing care of their patients according to the current ward management methodology.
12. **Evaluate** the patient's nursing care after each structured meeting – and **re-sign and re-date**. When changes have been made to the plan these must be re-authorised, signed and dated within 72 hours at the latest.
13. **Have a structured meeting** at agreed times with each patient **at least** every two days.
14. **Record the meeting** on a named nurse record sheet.

Reprinted from Dargan, R. (1997) *The Named Nurse in Practice*, copyright 1997, by permission of the publisher W B Saunders

Case/care management

Care management (Figure 5.5) is the activity of organising and managing the health and social provision for individuals where multi-disciplinary teams are involved but it is not a term that has been universally accepted in Britain. Case management is a term that has been brought over from the USA and often the phrase reflects the same ideas and is used interchangeably with care management. In Britain, the latter is preferable as the former reflects a demeaning 'person management'. The White Paper 'Caring for People' (Department of Health and Social Security 1989) identified the area of care management for health and social care needs and the policy document 'Community care in the next decade and beyond' (Department of Health 1990a) defined the processes of care management as:

- assessment of user's circumstances including support
- design of agreed care packages
- implementation and monitoring of agreed package.

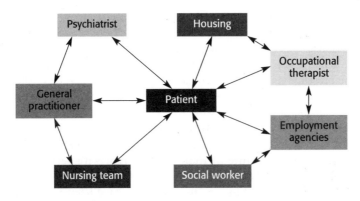

Figure 5.5 Case/care management

The internal market was the underlying concept of the NHS and Community Care Act 1990. The government of the day created the division between purchasers and providers of care in a market-like fashion, which also separated out health and social care. This was aimed at bringing about a division between care managers who were assessing needs and those providing care.

Ross and Mackenzie (1996) have highlighted the principles of care management as:

- an approach to assessment based on needs rather than services available
- a framework of locally determined objectives and priorities
- partnership among agencies
- partnership with client and carer
- information, monitoring, quality assurance and review.

Care management highlighted the need for a care manager. There were debates as to whether the care manager was distinctly different from a key worker in care. Ross and Mackenzie (1996) defined the care manager as 'Any practitioner who undertakes all or most of the core tasks of care management, who may also carry budgetary responsibility but is not involved in any direct service provision.' Community psychiatric nurses and district nurses were felt to be the best people to work as care managers because of their knowledge of the complex needs of their clients. These clients/patients were often the elderly or people with severe mental health problems. However, nurses acting as key workers were not always accepted. Management of community care had

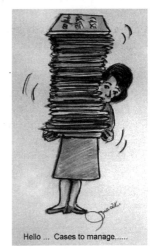

Hello ... Cases to manage......

its own difficulties. The pressure to move patients from hospital-based resources to community-based resources and therefore divide care into health-based or social-based provision was a feature of the government changes. Beds for the elderly and mentally ill were scaled down and the benefit to the health budget was that social care provision could be means-tested. This meant that care management was proving difficult due to inabilities to acquire resources for acute situations.

The ability of nurses to take on the purchasing of services was limited because of their employment conditions and it was considered that they had conflicts of interests because of their involvement with service provision. Therefore it was often seen as a role more easily taken on by social services. Nurses who were involved in care management have been in pilot schemes (Kent, Darlington and Gateshead) which were aimed at reducing the numbers of frail elderly people entering institutional care. These schemes included case finding, screening, needs assessment, planning and review as well as resource management. Studies of these schemes have demonstrated improvements in care quality and client satisfaction (Bergen 1992, Challis *et al.* 1989).

Care programme approach

The care programme approach was first introduced in 1991 specifically for the needs of people with complex mental health problems. North *et al.* (1993) noted that there were differences between care management (CM) and the care programme approach (CPA) which were not always understood.

The DoH circular HC (90) 23 identifies elements of care programmes:

1. Systematic arrangements for assessing health care needs of patients who could potentially be treated in the community and for regular review of those being treated in the community.
2. Systematic arrangements agreed with social service authorities for assessing and regularly reviewing what social care such patients need, to give them the opportunity of benefiting from treatment in the community.
3. Effective systems for ensuring that agreed health and, where necessary, social care services are provided to those patients who can be treated in the community.
4. Inter-professional collaboration was emphasised as well as patient and carer involvement.
5. Where a patient's minimum health or social care needs for treatment in the community cannot be met, in-patient treatment should be offered or continued.

What do you think some of the problems are with this process in serving the needs of patients with complex mental health needs?

Patients with complex mental health needs do not always feel that they are ill. Their health problems are often linked with housing and employment difficulties. They often have difficulties in communicating with family, friends, the wider community and helping agencies, even to the point of sometimes believing that they are being victimised. In trying to help these people there may be conflicts of interests between the patient/client, their family, the community and other professionals. The 'revolving door' scenario often meant that institutional care was unable to make any long-term plans due to limited bed space and only acute episodes were dealt with. The appointment of a key worker is still considered necessary to attempt overcome these problems. The key worker is seen as the professional who maintains contact with the client/patient on a regular basis in the community and is responsible for monitoring and implementing the care plans agreed. They have the problem of negotiating budgetary resources for individuals with the care managers who were interested in serving the needs of a defined community with a limited budget. North *et al.* (1993) identified factors that affected the successful implementation of the care programme approach in the community:

- lack of leadership in developing the approach
- complexity and bureaucracy of care management processes
- policy-making time and effort overtook the running of procedures
- need for better training to clarify roles for a collaborative approach
- in-patient resources were dwindling, forcing discharge into the community before the planning process and resources could be recognised; this meant the 'revolving door' of patients coming into and going out of acute care without long-term plans being made.

Within the next decade or so, changes in provision for patients with continuing problems will be problematic due to the need for integration of health and social care divisions.

Nursing Development Unit

The first documented Nursing Development Unit (NDU) in England, where primary nursing was the method of organising and delivering care, was in a small community hospital at Burford, Oxfordshire. From the late 1970s to the mid-1980s, the traditional ethos of working was being challenged and the emergence of a 'new nursing' was springing up, as nurses and patients found the benefit in a patient-centred approach. Also, major reorganisations in the NHS, such as those resulting from the recommendation of the Griffiths Report (Griffiths 1983), impacted on the role of nursing within management and power debates between nursing and 'management' became evident. Nurses wanted to maintain control of their own care environments so the concept of NDUs emerged out of these power struggles. McFarlane (1980) argued that there was a need to move away from the medical model of care which could be seen as:

Diagnosis → Treatment → Cure

to a nurse-led model:

Assessment (of self-care disabilities) → Help → Self care

The Oxford Nursing Unit, consisting of a purely nursing-led environment, became established in 1985 in an acute hospital. It was a very innovative, controlled experiment involving patients who had fractured femurs, in that there were no uniforms, the daily routines were patient-led with open visiting and nurses and patients sat down together for meals. Self-medication was encouraged and complementary therapy was practised. The nurses made improvement changes themselves, as part of a bottom-up management approach.

There were, however, problems with the research methodology (see Table 5.5) but the outcome was that the nurse-led care showed positive effects on patient satisfaction, recovery and mortality.

Table 5.5 The Hawthorne effect

Mayo, an American psychologist, looked at work groups at the Hawthorne Factory of Western Electric in Chicago in the 1920s. He observed the work of the employees and changed their working conditions e.g. more rest periods, various lighting and music conditions and various patterns of working. He found that there was an improvement in productivity after each change. However, productivity still improved when conditions reverted to their original state.

He reached the conclusion that:

● people behave differently when they are being observed
● productivity increased when employees became more involved and had attention paid to them
● the productivity improvement was not short-lived
● work groups organise themselves to suit the group norms rather then what management expects.

Write down what you think the Hawthorne Effect was at the Burford NDU.

At Burford, the fact that the research on nursing practice was being implemented meant that the nurses went out of their way to reflect a good level of nursing professionalism. It was this focus on practice and involvement of the nurses that led to an increase in patient satisfaction rather than the different way of organising the care delivery. However, the nursing morale was raised, and the good ideas generated needed to be captured and further research was instigated. NDUs are now not simply thought of in terms of concrete units, departments or wards. Nursing is now seen to be much broader – it takes place in homes, clinics, factories, schools, offices and during transportation. Nursing development is now about teams of people who are willing to net-work and who have a real desire to develop and change nursing practice. A 'bottom-up' approach to change is a value that underpins any development, even in creating an NDU. It was Salvage and Wright (1995) who felt that NDUs should focus on the following principles:

1. Nursing as a therapy.
2. The value of autonomy in pursuing goals.
3. A clinical base and a size that is manageable.
4. Use of a bottom-up approach to change.
5. The development of a shared culture.
6. The development of a nursing model.
7. A research-based exploration, application, dissemination and evaluation.
8. Clinical leadership and new nursing roles.
9. Patient empowerment and patient-centred care.
10. Multi-disciplinary partnership.
11. Equality in caring.
12. Organisational support and financial resources.
13. Staff development.

Burke (1998) highlighted the notion that NDUs encompassed the idea of empowerment. She considered that it was all right for nursing team members to be allowed to make mistakes and that criticism and disciplinary action should now be turned into support and staff development of individuals. This would in turn lead to individuals taking on more responsibility rather than less through a culture of fear.

What clinical areas, if any, in your Trust are designated as an NDU?

Conclusion

This chapter has given you an insight into the incremental changes in nurs-ing practice, examining the features that have been influential in the change process related to the delivery of care from the 1940s to the present day. However, it must be recognised that although there have been ongoing changes, early practices are not without value. Indeed, they must be seen in the context of a variety of practice environments and conditions, e.g. task allocation within an emergency situation where control and stability are of the essence.

The word 'change' is emotive and requires people to think about the values they had in the past and the way they have practised. Historically some nurses, midwives and health visitors have resisted change because it has been enforced through a 'top-down' approach rather than the more acceptable drive from the ground level. By being aware of the strengths and weaknesses of nursing structures, nurses can have more control over their role in care improvements, thus enhancing quality.

Summary of key points

This chapter has looked at the various ways that nursing has been organised in the pursuit of efficiency. Improvements are related to effectiveness, efficiency and economy.

- **Task allocation:** Focused on an efficient way of breaking the work down into tasks. Each staff member has particular skills and levels of competencies and these are matched to the tasks. It is still very useful today in cases of emergencies and staff shortages.

- **Team nursing:** Relates to nursing or midwifery staff working as a defined group to look after a set number of patients with an emphasis on patient allocation and total patient care.

- **Primary nursing:** Focused on the autonomy and responsibility of one nurse managing the total care of a patient.

- **Case/care management:** Looked at the value of multi-agency team working in the community.

- **Care programme approach:** Highlighted the value and problems of mult-agency team working in meeting complex mental health needs.

- **Nursing development units:** Focused on the development of a total nursing care philosophy and its impact on improving care delivery.

References

Audit Commission (1992) *Homeward Bound*, Audit Commission

Bergen A (1992) Case management in community care, concepts, practices and implications for nursing, *Journal of Advanced Nursing* **17**, 1106–13

Burke W (1998) The interview, *Nursing Management* **4** (8), 14–17

Challis D, Darton R, Johnson L, Stone M, Traske K and Wall B (1989) *Supporting Frail Elderly People at Home: The Darlington Community Care Project*, Canterbury Personal Social Services Research Unit: Kent University.

Clark J E, Copcutt L (eds)(1997) *Management for Nurses and Health Care Professionals*, Churchill Livingstone

Dargan R (1997) *The Named Nurse in Practice*, Baillière Tindall

Department of Health (1987) *Promoting Better Health – The Government's Programme for Improving Primary Health Care*, HMSO

Department of Health (1990a) *Community Care in the Next Decade and Beyond*, HMSO

Department of Health (1990b) *The NHS and Community Care Act*, HMSO

Department of Health (1991) *The Patient's Charter*, HMSO

Department of Health (1993) *New World, New Opportunities*, HMSO

Department of Health (1996) *Primary Care, Delivering the Future*, HMSO

Department of Health and Social Security (1989) *Caring for People*, HMSO

Duberley J (1977) How will the change strike me and you?, *Nursing Times*, **73** (45), 1736–8

Ersser S, Turton E (1991) *Primary Nursing in Perspective*, Scutari Press

Griffiths R (1983) *NHS Management Inquiry*, DHSS

Health Visitors Association (1996) *Integrated Nursing Team – Initial Information*, Professional Briefing, HVA

McFarlane J K (1980) *The Multi-Disciplinary Team*, King's Fund

Mitchell J R A (1984) Is nursing any business of doctors? A simple guide to the nursing process, *British Medical Journal*, **288**: 218–19

Neuman B (1982) *The Neuman Systems Model*, Appleton Century Crofts

North C, Ritchie J and Ward K (1993) *Factors Influencing the Implementation of Care Programme Approach*, HMSO

Orem D (1980) *Nursing – Concepts and Principles* (2nd edn) Little, Brown

Pearson A and Vaughan B (1986) *Nursing Models for Practice*, Heinemann

Peplau H E (1952) *Interpersonal Relations in Nursing*, Putnams

Roper N, Logan W and Tierney A (1981) *The Elements of Nursing*, Churchill Livingstone

Ross F and Mackenzie A (1996) *Nursing in Primary Health Care – Policy into Practice*, Routledge

Roy C (1976) *Introduction to Nursing: An Adaptation Model*, Prentice Hall

Salvage J and Wright S (1995) *Nursing Development Units*, Scutari Press

Tingle J (1993) Legal and professional implications of the named nurse concept, *British Journal of Nursing*, **2**(9), 480–2

UKCC (1992) *Code of Professional Conduct*, UKCC

van der Peet R (1995) *The Nightingale Model of Nursing*, Campion Press

Vestal K W (1987) *Nursing Management: Concepts and Issues* (2nd edn) Lippincott

Further reading

Aggleton P and Chalmers H (1986) *Nursing Models and the Nursing Process*, Macmillan

Binnie A and Tichen A (1999) *Freedom to Practice*, Butterworth Heinemann

Bull J (1998) Integrated nursing: a review of the literature, *British Journal of Nursing*, **3** (3), 124–9

Dargan R (1997) *The Named Nurse in Practice*, Baillière Tindall

Dunne L (ed.)(1991) *How Many Nurses Do I Need? A Guide to Resource Management Issues*, Wolfe Publishing

Ersser S and Tutton E (eds) (1991) *Primary Nursing in Perspective*, Scutari Press

Gould D (1988) *Nurses: The Inside Story of the Nursing Profession*, Unwin Paperbacks

Hart C (1994) *Behind the Mask: Nurses, Their Unions and Nursing Policy*, Baillière Tindall

Johns C (1994) *The Burford NDU Model – Caring in Practice*, Blackwell Science

Kendrick K, Weir P and Rosser E (1995) *Innovations in Nursing Practice*, Edward Arnold

Kenworthy N, Snowley G and Gilling C (1992) *Common Foundation Studies in Nursing*, Churchill Livingstone

Kershaw B and Salvage J (1986) *Models for Nursing*, Wiley

Lawler E and Porter L (1967) Antecedent attitudes of effective managerial perform-ance, *Organisational Behaviour and Human Performance*, **2**, 122–42

Leigh A and Maynard M (1995) *Leading Your Team: How to Involve and Inspire Teams*, Nicholas Brealey Publishing

Manthey M (1980) *The Practice of Primary Nursing*, Blackwell Scientific

McDermot G (1998) The care programme approach: a patient perspective, *Nursing Times*, **94** (8), 57–9

Nichol L H (ed.) (1986) *Perspectives on Nursing Theory*, Scott, Foreman

Pearson A (1988) *Primary Nursing*, Chapman & Hall

Reed J and Ground I (1997) *Philosophy of Nursing*, Edward Arnold

Rolfe G and Fulbrook P (1998) *Advanced Nursing Practice*, Butterworth Heinemann

Royal College of Nursing (1993) *Refusal to Nurse: Guidance for Nurses*, RCN

Rumbold G C (1995) *Management Skills for Community Nurses*, Central Health Studies

Welsh Institute for Health and Social Care/University of Glamorgan (1998) *Healthcare Futures 2010*, UKCC

Wright S (1998) *Changing Nursing Practice* (2nd edn) Edward Arnold

6

Leadership in health care

By the end of this chapter you will have had the opportunity to:

- define leadership, its meaning and importance
- discuss the value of various theories of leadership
- examine leadership as an aspect of behaviour
- evaluate a variety of leadership approaches
- critically discuss leadership in health care.

Introduction

When thinking about leaders in health care, we may initially identify with people like Florence Nightingale (1820–1910) and Mary Seacole (1805–1881) who did much for *caring* through their own pursuit of improving standards and acting as a role model in the health care work they did. But what about today? Why do we need leaders in nursing, midwifery and health visiting? Maybe because there is such a large number of nurses, midwives and health visitors throughout the country and also throughout the world and they all need to see a purpose in the work they do. Maybe, more importantly, the world of today is going through dramatic social change. Day-to-day change is also affected by the impact of what is known as the 'information revolution' on our everyday life, which is changing our daily work and home practices.

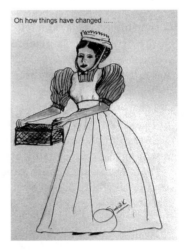

Oh how things have changed .....

What 'informational' changes can you think of?

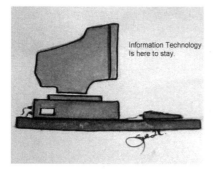

Information Technology
Is here to stay.

You may well have thought about the coming of digital television and the use of the personal computer and the mobile telephone but there is also the increasing access to the World Wide Web, the electronic technologies in hospitals and health centres and the globalisation of industry in general. We should not forget, however, that this revolution has often made the gap wider between 'those that have' and 'those that have not'. This can be taken in the context of the poor and rich in a certain country but also between countries, e.g. the campaign for obliteration of the Third World debt.

So why are leaders needed in this changing world? Well, it would be easy to say 'to maintain the status quo' and feel that we have no need to move with the times as caring never changes... but we know it does! As health care expectations rise and technological advancement increases, nurses, midwives and health visitors need to be ready for the changes in the twenty-first century so that they have the knowledge and skills demanded of them. Leaders are therefore needed to guide the way forward.

Concept and roles of leadership

Leadership is seen as an elusive concept. Indeed, leading writers cannot agree on the nature or essential characteristics of leadership but offer a variety of definitions. Bernhart and Walsh (1990, p. 16) identify leadership as a process that is 'used to move a group towards goal setting and goal achievement ... and can be learned'. Stewart (1996, p. 3) cites Field-Marshall Lord Slim who said that it is 'of the spirit, compounded of personality and vision'. She goes on to say that it is about discovering the route ahead and encouraging and inspiring others to follow. So is it, perhaps, about how far they see ahead and how they use their personality to show others the way? Rafferty (1993, pp. 3–4), in discussing leaders as people, felt that they 'have that combination of conceptual ability, vision that is driven ... from an emotional front and some practical ability to achieve that vision'. She then goes on to say that they

> inspire you and whom others will follow but who will trust you. They will trust in your integrity.... Leaders care for the people they are leading/serving. Leaders try to strengthen and promote these people.... They facilitate and help and encourage and praise.

Mullins (1999, p. 253) indicates that Lord Sieff (Sieff 1991) maintained that:

Leadership is vitally important at all levels ... the moral and intellectual ability to visualise and work for what is best for the company and its employees ... to be effective leadership has to be seen, and it is best seen in action.

So, while there would appear to be no agreed definition of what a leader is, it can be seen that leaders do have a set of roles that seem to be universally accepted. They include:

- periodic review of induction and orientation programmes for new staff
- generate enthusiasm in employees related to organisational goals
- clarify organisation and unit goals
- infuse team spirit
- be a role model
- direction giving in times of crisis
- encourage mentorship
- encourage and support professional development
- support staff during personal and professional difficulties
- assist in the development of coping strategies.

You may be able to think of others. However, when discussing the roles and responsibilities of the 'leader' it is often the 'role model' and 'directional' elements that are focused upon to the detriment of staff support and other components.

Leaders and managers do not always equate to the same person. A manager is formally appointed to a designated role whereas a leader may emerge from anywhere within a team. Many leaders act in a role that has never been clearly identified, established or defined.

Vision, goals and direction

A 'vision' and a 'direction' for the team working together are therefore seen as important. Organisations and teams may be about learning to take a vision forward to 'fit' in with a changing environment. In today's health service this may be about keeping a customer/patient focus, continuous and speedy adaptation, devolved decision making, enabling structures, rewarding flexibility and a learning and reflexive climate (Holdaway and Kogan 1997, Pedlar 1997). It is important when nursing, midwifery and health visitor leaders emerge that they have a vision and can then share future goals with the team of people involved.

- What does this mean for nurses, midwives and health visitors?
- What is vision?

A vision could be said to involve ideals and principles and be described as: a living picture of the future desirable state combining:

- thought content
- emotional value and
- moral symbolic value. (Burnside 1991, p. 194)

These are admirable qualities, but will they take a team forward? Shirley (1991) pointed to the dangers of people planning by vision alone and to the need for:

- good analysis
- financial awareness
- the spread of energy and motivation throughout a whole organisation

to support the 'dream'. Further to this, Sir Adrian Cadbury highlighted that organisations should be judged by their actions, not just their pious statements of intent (Silva 1977).

Leadership theories

The concept of leadership, however, will be different things to different people and therefore may well be defined depending on the various perspectives on leadership. There have been varying ways put forward for classifying leadership theories (Rafferty 1993, Mullins 1999) but it may be useful to look at leadership in the following forms to combine these ideas:

- leadership as a collection of personal characteristics or traits
- leadership as a function within an organisation
- leadership as an effect on group behaviour
- leadership as a culture.

Leadership as a collection of personal characteristics or traits

These theories were popular at the beginning of the century and focused on the idea of some universal traits of leaders. This was seen as useful in order to identify potential leaders for the future. So what do *you* think about effective leaders? What characteristics do you think they need? Are they different from those that were needed one hundred years ago?

> Write down any leadership characteristics that you think are important from what you have experienced or have heard about.

You may have a list that includes the following: someone who knows what has got to be done; who gets things done; who is a good communicator; who is admirable; who is a good persuader; who is good at bringing in change. You may, however, have found this difficult as the way that people lead varies and sometimes it is hard to identify characteristics that they all share. This may be because, in different contexts, leaders require different attributes.

Marquis and Huston (1996) (Table 6.1) also identify certain characteristics of leaders in terms of their intelligence, personality and abilities. However, in the mid-1940s the research was inconclusive and contradictory in relation to evidence about traits, especially as the relationship between leaders and the context of the situation were seen as more important. Trait theory has also been criticised because it does not seem to take account of the organisational culture and may even negate the part that social class, gender and race inequalities play in maintaining the status quo in leadership positions. There are, however, remnants of trait theory in trying to set desirable attributes and competencies for positions in nursing, midwifery and health visiting (person specification, job description and grade description will be examined in Chapter 12). The qualities or traits approach does give rise to some questions such as whether leaders are born or made, together with whether leadership is an art or a science. Whatever your feelings on this, for leadership to be effective you do need to apply special skills and techniques.

Table 6.1 Leadership characteristics

Intelligence	Personality	Abilities
Knowledge	Adaptability	Able to enlist cooperation
Judgement	Creativity	Interpersonal skills and tact
Decisiveness	Cooperativeness	Diplomacy
Oral fluency	Alertness	Prestige
	Self-confidence	Social participation
	Personal integrity	
	Emotional balance and control	
	Non-conformity	
	Independence	

From Marquis, B. L. and Huston, L. J. (1996) *Leadership Roles and Management Functions in Nursing: Theory and Applications, 2nd Edition* (Lippincott Williams and Wilkins).

Leadership as a function within an organisation

Here the emphasis is on what leaders actually do and relates to the function that a particular leader plays in an organisation. Adair (1979) approached effective leadership with the idea that in action-centred leadership there was an ability to meet three functions:

1. To achieve the required task(s).
2. To maintain the team.
3. To meet the needs of individual team members.

His three-sphere model highlights the overlapping areas of functions (Figure 6.1).

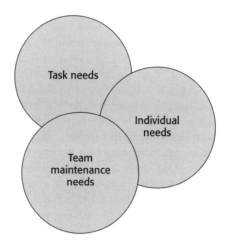

Figure 6.1 Interaction of needs within the group.
After Adair, J. (1979)

How could this model of leadership apply in nursing, midwifery and health visiting?

It can be argued that, historically, nursing fits into this model well (Chapter 5). When examining achievement of the *required tasks*, it is easy to see that if patient care is related to specific tasks (Chapter 5) then the planning of work revolves around a variety of areas: the individual task; the allocation of resources to achieve that task; and the organisation of skill mix in order to ensure the quality of performance. It is about the delivery of physical care in an effective and efficient manner and may not consider the psychological needs of the patient/client. Leaders in health care have to think about the type of work and jobs that have to be done for the health service to survive. When you go onto a ward in the morning, there are certain tasks that have to be organised and dealt with.

Can you think of any examples?

There are patients who will be hungry and will need to be offered breakfast. They or their relatives will expect to see their doctors in order to find out whether there are any results from diagnostic tests, so doctors' rounds have to be organised. There may be patients who will need to be prepared for surgery, X-ray, MRI scans, etc. Some patients will need to be admitted and some discharged from hospital. The various patients' needs will have to be addressed in order of priority. In the community there are similar tasks that have to be done such as the administration of referrals, telephone contacts, visits to book, patient/client visits to make and clinics to run as well as liaison meetings. Filling up with petrol is also a task that has to be fitted in! Managing and leading teams will require leaders to think about how these activities will be achieved:

- setting and achieving goals and objectives to get the required work done
- communicating goals and objectives to the rest of the team
- defining the tasks to meet the objectives
- planning the work
- bargaining for and mobilising resources, e.g. beds, linen, people
- delegating the work, organising responsibilities and supporting the team
- monitoring performance and quality management
- reviewing progress.

However, when we consider the *maintenance of the team* then we must consider team building, recognising training needs and communication systems within the group (Chapter 5). Teams require leaders and followers. These may not always be the same people as roles may change. The people in the team, however, have to have the right skills, knowledge and attitudes for the tasks to be completed if the team is to be successful. The following are issues for any team leader:

- team building and encouraging a team spirit
- encouraging a working cohesive team unit
- setting standards and professional behaviour
- setting up systems of communication within the team
- training and developing the team
- delegating and developing others.

The third element, *meeting the needs of individual team members*, requires the leader to give attention to personal needs or problems while giving praise and status to the individual. Again, professional development and training have to be recognised in order to raise the quality of care delivery. Team individuals will have personal needs as well. They will come to work for a variety of reasons, besides money. They will want to be valued and developed within the working team. Leaders may well need to think about the following:

- appraising and listening to the needs of individuals
- attending to personal problems
- giving praise and status to individuals
- reconciling conflicts between team needs and individual needs

- training and developing individuals
- clinical supervision and reflective practices.

The action by the leader to ensure that all this occurs will affect one or both of the other areas of need. The ideal is, of course, the position in the centre where all three areas are integrated and the needs are adequately met and the team or group is satisfied. Adair (1990) more recently stated that the future requires leaders with:

- direction
- team building capacity
- creativity.

This is interesting because it relates to the fact that traditional nursing leadership does not necessarily fit in with the complexity of contemporary health care. With teams that reflect a broader range of skill mix, with increasing demands of patients/clients and increasingly complex needs, nurse leaders need to be more flexible and creative in their problem solving than they ever have been before.

Leadership as an effect on group behaviour

The way an individual leads within an organisation or a team has been seen in terms of their style of behaviour. One way of looking at the leadership style is in connection with the power that a managerial leader exerts over the subordinates in a team.

- *The autocratic or authoritarian style*: the leader exercises ultimate power in decision making and controls the rewards and punishments for the subordinates in conforming to their decisions.
- *The democratic and participative style*: the leader encourages all members of the team to interact and to contribute to the decision making process.
- *The laissez-faire style*: the leader *conscientiously* makes the decision to pass the focus of power on to the subordinate members in genuine *laissez-faire* style. This is distinct from abdication or 'non-leadership' when the 'leader' refuses to make any decisions.

Several behavioural researchers, whose work has influenced management perspectives, are worthy of note here. McGregor (1987), an American psychologist of the 1960s, looked at employee types and identified that there were two types of employee behaviour (Table 6.2):

- theory X behaviour
- theory Y behaviour.

Table 6.2 Theory X and theory Y: employee behaviour.

Theory X employee behaviour (resulting from autocracy)	Theory Y behaviour (resulting from participatory leadership)
People hate work	People like work
People have to be forced to work	People drive themselves to work effectively
People prefer to be told what to do	People will take the initiative if given the opportunity
People are selfish and have no interest in the organisation	People will commit themselves to the organisation if it is beneficial

Adapted from Macgregor (1987)

These assumed behaviours were considered the *result*, not the *cause*, of the style of management used. If theory Y behaviours were required of employees, then the style of leadership required would be less autocratic and more participative. Linked to McGregor's idea was that of Tannenbaum and Schmidt (1983) who first recognised that managers needed varying mixtures of autocracy and democracy depending on the situation. They suggested that leadership could be seen as a continuum from *boss-centred* to *subordinate-centred*. The former relates to the X theory and the latter relates to the Y theory of McGregor. Blake and Mouton (1985) also compared leadership styles in terms of two dimensions:

1. Concern for the task.
2. Concern for people.

Have you met professionals who are good in one of these areas but not in the other?

It is a very special health professional who is always able to come to terms with managing these two areas equally. Blake and Mouton describe these two dimensions on a Leadership Grid® (Figure 6.2) and highlight five types of managerial leader on an axial basis:

1. The impoverished manager (1,1) has low concern for the task and for people.
2. The authority-compliance manager (9,1) has high concern for the task and low concern for people.
3. The country club manager (1,9) has low concern for the task but high concern for people.
4. The middle-of-the-road manager (5,5) has moderate concern for the task and moderate concern for people.
5. The team manager (9,9) as an ideal has high concern for the task and for people.

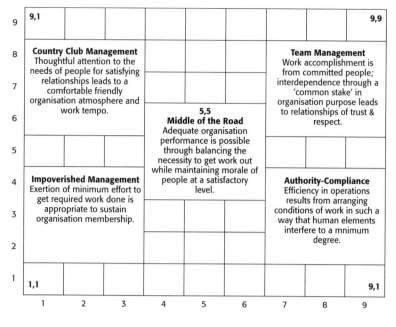

Figure 6.2 The Leadership Grid®
From Blake R and Mouton J (1985)

Leadership as a part of culture formation

These theories are more recent and combine views from any of the others above. They show leadership in the context of changing cultures and dynamics especially prevalent within different health care environments. Schein (1985) felt that leadership needs to be seen in context and the culture of that context is important: 'Leadership is entwined with culture formation.' The type of leadership required in health care is one that therefore fits with the culture of the organisation in which that health care is delivered. Schein (1992) defined organisational culture as:

> The pattern of basic assumptions that a given group has invented, discovered or developed in learning to cope with its problems of external adaptation and internal integration ... and therefore taught to new members as the correct way to perceive, think and feel in relation to those problems.

This can be seen within the organisational culture of a hospital or community placement and also within university life. Induction at the start of a new course and meeting up with lecturers, mentors and other students on the course as well as people who have nearly finished their course integrate us into what is expected in terms of our behaviour within the university. During our first clinical placements we note the way other professionals behave and react to patients, clients and their relatives. Schein (1992) also argued that there was a need to understand the dynamic and evolutionary forces that govern cultural change, which has to be taken on board in light of the new culture of our own professional education and training.

Circumstantial theories

These theories made their mark in the 1960s with the idea that leadership is more than the qualities held by the leaders themselves. Leaders develop according to the demands and circumstances of the situation. Fiedler (1967) identified that no one particular style of leadership meets the needs of every situation and so developed a contingency model. In order to measure attitudes of the leader Fiedler developed a scale that measured the relationship between the leader and another person with whom they would work. The questionnaire contains up to twenty items ranging from pleasant/unpleasant, helpful/unhelpful and distant/close to open/guarded. Each item has a ranking of 1 to 8 with 8 being the most favourable and 1 being the least favourable. Fiedler's original interpretation of this was that if the leader scored highly then the indication was good in terms of interpersonal relationships with the team. Conversely, if the score was low then the leader was seen to derive most satisfaction from knowing that a specific task had been completed rather than considering the implication of relationships within that achievement. However, as a piece of scientific research this has been challenged over the years. Fiedler's work has been subjected to much criticism but it is worth recognising the contribution that it has made to gauging leader effectiveness. It is, however, arguable as to its real value as the best style of leadership in any situation is a variable in itself and dependent on the environmental situation.

Taking and applying this theory to nursing, midwifery and health visiting, it may be seen that within an emergency situation the autocratic style will be adopted. This directional approach may not be liked or appreciated by all the members of the team but it will be the most effective way of handling the situation. A score following an incident may be lower than at other times. Of course this does not necessarily mean that the leader was wrong in adopting that approach but, human nature being what it is, not everyone likes to be told what to do.

Transformational theories

These theories are based on the idea that leaders are people who motivate others to perform by encouraging them to see a vision and change in their perception of reality. They are seen as committed individuals with long-term vision and a need to empower others and who are interested in the consequences. They use:

- charisma
- individualised consideration
- intellectual stimulation to produce greater effort, effectiveness and satisfaction in followers
- inspiration through symbols (Bass and Avolio 1990).

Burns (1978) identifies that the transforming process is one in which leaders and followers raise *each other* to higher levels of morals and motivation, so values such as liberty, peace, equality and humanitarianism are often emphasised rather than values based on individual benefits. However, it has been noted that transformational leaders can have the potential for accruing a good deal of control and power, which can lead to the exploitation of large numbers of followers. Great leaders can be seen as very positive, such as:

- Mohandas Gandhi
- Martin Luther King
- John Kennedy
- Nelson Mandela.

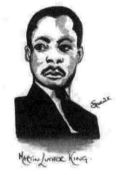

Martin Luther King

However, there may be transformational leaders who are portrayed in a negative light:

- Adolf Hitler
- Charles Manson
- David Koresh.

Other criticisms of transformational leaders may be that they tend to focus on the bigger issues of life and because of their high visibility are unwilling to spend time with facilitating change. Thus to followers, leaders may be seen as autocratic; success is often about the detail of getting things done. The old adage may be appropriate: 'The devil is in the detail'.

Contractual theories

These theories are known as transactional leadership theories and are often contrasted to transformational leadership theories. Contractual or transactional leaders benefit from stable environments. Similarly, leaders and followers will be mutually satisfied with the relationship. There are some that want to lead and there are others who require leadership.

Bass (1985) defined transactional leadership as having:

- rewards and incentives to influence motivation
- the ability for the leader to monitor and correct subordinates in order to work effectively
- an explicit promise of tangible benefits for followers
- an ideological appeal.

Marquis and Huston (1996) identified the characteristics of a transactional leader as follows:

- focuses on management tasks
- caretakes
- uses trade-offs to meet goals
- shared values not identified
- examines causes
- uses contingency rewards.

It could be that through personal mastery, group synergy, learning and sustainable development, this new leadership will emerge. Bennis *et al.* (1994) and Malby (1994) support this view and identify that the time is right for leading in this way within a framework of increased accountability. Scott (1998) points to the value of improving relationships between settings, process-based skills and professional judgement for the future of nursing leadership.

Leadership and the future

Professional leadership in the twenty-first century will be essential in order to meet the demands for health care in the future. New roles and expectations will drive nursing into a more prominent position. Nurse prescribing, nurse consultant-led clinics and nurses managing doctors are signs of this challenge for nurses. Practice leadership as well as educational and research leadership will be required by the profession to respond to the demands of society. Indeed, *A Vision for the Future* (Department of Health/NHS Executive 1993) recognised the need for leadership at all levels of professional life. Leadership for a changing world will require new skills. Kanter (1991) identifies specific skills:

- self-mastery
- strategic visioning
- continual learning
- creator of partnerships
- team facilitator.

Multi-agency teams will be a feature of the future and they too will require appropriate leadership. Mintzberg *et al.* (1998, p. 588) highlighted that vision, shared ideals, creation of organisational pride and developing environments for energies and innovation are considered to be essential attributes of leadership. They also identify that a unique and essential leadership function is to build an organisation's culture and shape its evolution. They go on to suggest that the leadership roles of designer, teacher and steward were required for contributing to leadership *in the past* but propose that new meanings will be needed for 'learning' organisations *of the future*. Will nurses, midwives and health visitors be able to rise to these demands? It is to be hoped that they will not accept the traditional 'follower' roles of the past. The following quote from Lao-Tsu (604–531 BC) is a useful ending for this chapter:

> As for the best leaders, the people do not notice their existence. The next best, the people honour and praise. The next, the people fear, and the next the people hate. When the best leader's work is done, the people say 'we did it ourselves!' (Robertson 1997, p. 278)

Conclusion

Throughout this chapter you have been asked to examine a variety of leadership theories and their relevance to the workplace today. This is often a difficult task because we do not tend to look at the theories; rather, we accept that some people are natural leaders while others are content to follow. It is important to recognise how you present yourself and how you have developed or will develop your preferred leadership style as you go through the course of study. By understanding the nature of leadership it becomes easier to develop your own individual style for given situations. As stated earlier, it comes naturally to some people whereas others have to work towards it.

Summary of key points

During this chapter we have examined a variety of factors related to leadership theory.

- **Concepts and roles:** Identified the need to have an idea about the overall need for leaders within the health service. Here we identified the rapid technological changes that are taking place within the health service and the effect they are having on patient care. It was also seen that there is no clear definition of what a leader is; rather, there was a general feeling that they would be a good 'role model'.

- **Vision, goal and direction:** Went on to examine the needs of common purpose in order to take the care provision forward.

- **Leadership theory:** identified a variety of leadership traits or characteristics, each of which was shown to have an effect on patient/client care provision.

- **Circumstantial theories:** Showed that the effectiveness of the leader was thought to correlate well with the situation or circumstances within which the leader was working.

- **Transformational theories:** Talked about the transforming process that some leaders demonstrate in either a positive or negative way.

- **Contractual/transactional theories:** Are often seen as being the opposite of transformational in order to offset the change process.

- **Leadership in the twenty-first century:** Was shown to be necessary in order to meet the demands of the future. Discussion took place related to the expanding role of the nurse leading to a stronger voice for nurses, midwives and health visitors.

References

Adair J (1979) *Action Centred Leadership*, Gower Press

Adair J (1990) *Great Leaders*, Brookwood Talbot, Adair Press

Bass B (1985) *Leadership and Performance Beyond Expectations*, New York, Free Press

Bass B and Avolio B J (1990) Developing transformational leadership: 1992 and beyond, *Journal of European Industrial Training*, **14**, 21–7

Bennis W, Parikh J and Leesom R (1994) *Beyond Leadership: Balancing Economics, Ethics and Ecology*, Blackwell

Bernhart L A and Walsh M (1990) *Leadership: The Key to the Professionalization of Nursing*, C V Mosby

Blake R R and Mouton J S (1985) *The Managerial Grid III*, Gulf Publishing

Burns J (1978) *Leadership*, Harper and Row

Burnside R (1991) Visioning: building pictures of the future, in Henry J and Walker D, *Managing Innovation*, Sage Publications/Open University

Department of Health/NHS Executive (1993) *A Vision for the Future*, HMSO

Fiedler F E (1967) *Theory of Leadership Effectiveness*, McGraw-Hill

Holdaway K and Kogan H (eds) (1997) *The Healthcare Management Handbook* (2nd edn) Institute of Health Services Management/Kogan Page

Kanter R M (1991) Change master skills: what it takes to be creative, in Henry J and Walker D (eds) (1991) *Managing Innovation*, Sage Publications/Open University

Malby R (1994) *The Challenges for Nursing and Midwifery in the 21st Century: A Briefing Document*, University of Leeds

Marquis B L and Huston C J (1996) *Leadership Roles and Management Functions in Nursing: Theory and Application* (2nd edn) Lippincott

McGregor D (1987) *The Human Side of Enterprise*, Penguin

Mintzberg H, Quinn J B and Ghoshal S (1998) *The Strategy Process*, Prentice Hall

Mullins L (1999) *Management and Organisational Behaviour* (5th edn) Pitman

Pedlar M (1997) *The Learning Company: A Strategy for Sustainable Development* (2nd edn) McGraw-Hill

Rafferty A (1993) Leading questions: a discussion paper on the issues of nurse leadership, King's Fund Centre

Robertson C (1997) *The Wordsworth Dictionary of Quotations*, Wordsworth Editions

Scott I (1998) Challenging the Future. *Nursing Management*, **4**(9) 18–21

Schein E H (1985) *Organizational Culture and Leadership*, Jossey-Bass

Schein E H (1992) Coming to a new awareness of organizational culture, in Salaman G (ed.) (1992) *Strategic Human Resource Management*, Sage Publications/Open University

Shirley S (1991) Corporate strategy and entrepreneurial vision, in Henry J and Walker D (1991) *Managing Innovation*, Sage Publications/Open University

Sieff M (Lord Sieff of Brimpton) (1991) *Management the Marks & Spencer Way*, Fontana Collins

Silva M C (1977) Philosophy, science and theory: interrelationships and implications for nursing research, *Image*, **9** (3), 59–63

Stewart R (1996) *Leading in the NHS: A Practical Guide* (2nd edn) Macmillan Business

Tannenbaum R and Schmidt W H (1983) How to choose a leadership pattern, *Harvard Business Review*, May–June, 162–80

Further reading

Ansoff H I (1969) *Business Strategy*, Penguin

Antobus S, Pickard D, Reed A and Sutton E (1999) Strategy of success, *Primary Health Care*, **9**(1), 8–12

Argyris C (1958) The organisation: what makes it healthy?, *Harvard Business Review*, **36**(6), 107–16

Daft R L (1989) *Organisational Theory and Design* (3rd edn) Mid-West Publishing

Department of Health (1997) *The New NHS: Modern and Dependable*, The Stationery Office

Drucker P (1989) *The Practice of Management*, Heinemann Professional

Drucker P (1992) The coming of the new organisation, in Salaman G (ed.)(1992) *Strategic Human Resource Management*, Sage Publications/Open University

Etzioni A (1975) *A Comparative Analysis of Complex Organisations* (rev. edn) Free Press

Girvin J (1998) *Leadership and Nursing*, Macmillan

Handy C (1991) *The Age of Unreason* (2nd edn), Century Business

Harrigan K R and Porter M E (1989) End-game strategies for declining industries, in Ash D and Bowman C (eds) *Readings in Strategic Management*, Macmillan/Open University

Johnson G and Scholes K (1989) *Exploring Corporate Strategy*, Prentice Hall

Mintzberg H (1989) in Open University (1993) B884 *Human Resource Strategies Block 2 Unit 3*, p. 26, Open University Press

Ouchi W G (1981) *Theory Z: How American Business Can Meet the Japanese Challenge*, Addison-Wesley

Pfeffer J and Salancik G R (1978) *The External Control of Organizations: A Resource Dependence Perspective*, Harper & Row

Sievers B (1993) *Work, Death and Life Itself: Essays on Management and Organization*, De Gruyter

Townsend R (1985) *Further Up the Organization*, Coronet Books

7

Management theory applied to health care

By the end of this chapter you will have had the opportunity to:

- consider the structure and function of organisations and the implications of nursing within an organisational framework
- describe the components of an organisation
- discuss which systems of management are appropriate to health care organisation and nursing management
- appreciate the importance of adopting a caring and positive approach to management in a 'people-centred' organisation
- discuss external influences on management systems
- make suggestions of criteria for the evaluation of managerial effectiveness.

Introduction

No single management theory provides all the answers but in order for you to function effectively it is vital that management theory is utilised in the health care setting and is understood. The main approaches to organisational structure and management, when examined in terms of their social context, demonstrate a progression in understanding the needs of people involved within that organisation. The main approaches to be discussed within this chapter are classical, human relations, systems and contingency and management by objectives.

When initially designing an organisation, decisions have to be made relating to its structure. Prior to the first Industrial Revolution (early nineteenth Century) traditional authority based on autocracy, hierarchy, rules and regulations was uppermost. Factory and mine owners wielded power over their employees by having control not only within the workplace but also over the often sparse living accommodation. Furthermore, usually the whole family worked for one master with linked business enterprises. Thus control was more far reaching, for if one member of the family was to find difficulty with the 'boss' then it might have repercussions for the others. So it can be seen that there was a set of rules that had to be adhered to. In some instances other forms of authority (charismatic and legal–rational) could be seen but they appear more in modern society where we comply with managers' wishes because of the authority and power they possess. This chapter will explore the use and effects of the main management theories in the context of health care provision.

Importance of management theory

In order to be an effective manager, or even to function effectively within an organisation, it is important to know why an organisation might function in a specific way. Miner (1980) makes the point that 'the more we know about organisations and their methods of operation, the better the chances of dealing effectively with them'. So it is necessary to view the different elements of an organisation in order to understand why it functions in a specific manner. It can also help to clarify how you might be expected to behave in a given situation in order to uphold the reputation of that organisation. Similarly, it may help us adopt management practices that, while 'old', might be the most appropriate for a given situation.

Purpose of organisations

Organisations exist to achieve a purpose through the cooperation of members of that organisation. The shape, structure and function changes in order to achieve what is set out in the organisational purpose. Organisations come in all forms, shapes and sizes.

Can you identify some organisation to which you belong?

You might have thought of quite a few, including professional organisations, leisure centres, hospitals, retail shops, schools, or you may attend/use various, airports, hotels, government departments, banks, and local authorities. Although the organisations you have highlighted might be different, they will all have four factors in common:

1. People.
2. Objectives/purpose.
3. Structure.
4. Application of some sort of management theory.

Mullins (2000) suggests that 'it is the interaction of *People* in order to achieve *Objectives* that are channelled and co-ordinated through *Structure* and directed and controlled by *Management* which contribute to the success of an organisation'. It can be seen, however, that within any organisation the formal structure coexists with the informal element. We all know of the efficiency, but not always accuracy, of the 'grapevine', i.e. the informal element.

Basic components of an organisation

Within any organisation there will be a variety of people but in the main they can be loosely divided into the people who undertake the work of providing the service and the managers who are concerned with supervision and coordination of the services offered. There are five basic components of an organisation which can be readily seen within health care provision and which interact with each other to ensure the smooth running of the service:

1. *Operational core*, which is concerned with direct performance of technical and productive operations (nurses; doctors; all staff involved in the delivery of care).
2. *Operational support*, concerned indirectly with technical and productive process but closely related to actual flow of work (quality control; works maintenance).
3. *Organisational support:* provision of services for whole organisation (occupational health; personnel; canteen services).
4. *Top management*, concerned with broad objectives and policy, strategic decisions, interactions with external environment (chief executive; Trust board).
5. *Middle management*, concerned with coordination and integration of activities; providing links with operational and organisational support staff and between operational core and top management (ward sister/charge nurse; directorate or divisional managers).

Figure 7.1 demonstrates the interaction among these five components and it can be seen that middle management is the linchpin that holds it all together, but we must recognise that each person has their place and without each other the organisation will not function effectively.

The structure of an organisation influences its culture. Organisational culture is made up of those symbolic elements and interactions that are unique to that organisation such as formal charts, rules and procedures. The stability of organisational structure and culture was a feature in the booming 1950s and 1960s but by the mid-1980s firms and businesses, including the health service, had to change to fit with the changing economics and environmental market lifestyle. The health service saw the impact of the reduction of student nurses through P2K, along with the growth of health care assistants, and these structural changes made a huge impact on the NHS culture as well. Burns and Stalker (1994) noted two different and polarised organisational systems in industry: the mechanistic cultural system and the organic cultural system. The mechanistic organisation is rigid and bureaucratic, and more suitable for stable conditions. It is characterised by:

- specialisation of tasks
- closely defined duties and responsibilities
- a clear hierarchical structure
- knowledge at the top
- instructional basis by superiors
- insistence on loyalty to the organisation.

The organic organisation is more fluid, which is more appropriate to changing conditions, and is characterised by:

- specialised knowledge and experience contributed to the tasks
- tasks adjusted and redefined
- knowledge located throughout the organisation
- importance and prestige attached to individual contribution
- network of control and authority
- communication based on information giving rather than instructions and decisions
- commitment to the tasks.

These models can be seen as characterising the NHS, which has changed from a mechanistic organisation in those early years to a more organic organisation today. The health service now relies less on hierarchical structures and other models of organisational structure can be more useful in seeing how it functions.

Atkinson (1984) described what is known as *the flexible firm* which helped with dealing with uncertainty in the workforce. He suggested that firms are really looking for three kinds of flexibility:

1. *Functional flexibility* allowing for rapid deployment of multi-skilled workers.
2. *Numerical flexibility* in order to restructure the organisation to match the demand for labour.
3. *Financial flexibility* in order that pay and other employment costs can reflect the supply and demand of labour.

Similarly, Handy (1989) identified a shamrock model of organisation life. The shamrock leaves were made up of the following:

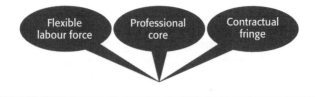

Jot down what kind of nursing, midwifery or health visiting staff you see in these group.

These two models highlight the difficulties of staffing in ward areas, community bases and nursing homes where there is a core group of regular permanent staff who work on both day and night shifts. There is also a group of bank staff (some of whom may also be permanent staff willing to take on an extra shift). There are also agency nurses who come in to fill the gaps in the workforce and who work on *ad hoc* contracts. This flexibility helps to cope with high demands being put on permanent staff. Students also add to this extra supply of staff but may not formally be regarded as staff.

The changing face of recruitment and retention means that there are generally fewer trained nurses than ever before and concern is rising that the number of core staff is continually decreasing in many clinical areas and this flexible workforce is increasing. What impact does this have on those who manage various care environments? Staff who work in clinical areas on a day-to-day basis will obviously require new, creative insight and leadership skills.

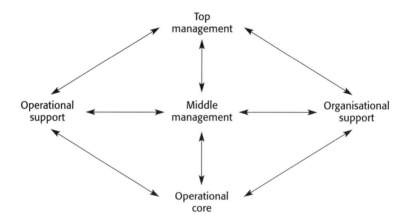

Figure 7.1 Interaction of five main managerial components

The formal and informal organisation

The nature of the formal organisation is normally dictated by the senior managers and may include such elements as the working environment, shift patterns and staff numbers. The informal organisation, on the other hand, exists within the formal structure in order to support people's social and psychological needs.

As we have seen, organisations exist to achieve their objectives; they do not exist to satisfy their employees' needs. Thus within any formal organisation there is an informal element that caters for more personal needs. Table 7.1 demonstrates some of the differences so, we can see that the features of the formal organisation include the following:

Table 7.1 Characteristics of the formal and informal organisation within the NHS

Characteristic	Formal organisation	Informal organisation
1. Structure		
A. Origin	Planned	Spontaneous
B. Rationale	Rationale	Emotional
C. Characteristics	Stable	Dynamic (ever changing)
2. Position terminology	Job	Role that may not be formally recognised
3. Goals	Profitability or service to society	Member satisfaction
4. Influence		
A. Base	Position	Personality
B. Type	Authority	Power
C. Flow	Top-down	Bottom-up
5. Control mechanisms	Threat of firing, demotion	Physical or social norms
6. Communication		
A. Channels	Formed channels	Grapevine
B. Networks	Well defined, follow formal lines	Poorly defined, cut across regular channels
C. Speed	Slow	Fast
D. Accuracy	High	Low
7. Charting the organisation	Organisation chart	Sociogram
8. Miscellaneous		
A. Individuals Included	All individuals work in the group	Only those 'acceptable'
B. Interpersonal relations	Prescribed by job description	Arise spontaneously
C. Leadership role	Assigned by organisation	Result of member agreement
D. Basis for interaction	Functional duties or position	Personal characteristics
E. Basis for attachment	Loyalty	Cohesiveness

From Gray J L and Starke F A (1984) *Organisational Behaviour: Concepts and Applications, 3rd Edition*. Reprinted by permission of Pearson Education, Inc.

- the planned coordination of the activities of a number of people for the achievement of some common, explicit purpose or goal
- difference between formal and informal organisation is a feature of the degree to which they are structured
- formal deliberately planned and created, and is concerned with the coordination of activities
- hierarchically structured, stated objectives, specification of tasks, defined relationships of authority and responsibility
- may have rules and regulations, standing orders, job description.

whereas the informal organisation includes:

- recognition that it arises from the interaction of people working within the organisation
- relationships that are undefined
- membership being spontaneous with varying degrees of involvement
- group relationships and norms of behaviour existing outside the organisation and these may be in conflict with the aims of the formal organisation.

Examining this in the context of the clinical environment, one can see that the wards and departments are heavily involved in the formal element of the organisation whereas informal organisation occurs within people, i.e. the support network for one another. Sometimes the informal organisation can be the largest element if its components were to be identified and plotted. Lysons (1997) likened these organisational elements to an iceberg where by far the largest part (the informal element) is hidden beneath the surface supporting that which can be seen (the tip of the formal iceberg). Within health service provision these two elements coexist. However, we have all experienced the workings of the informal approach via rumour which often initiates change within work practices (see Chapter 8).

The classical approach to management

The classical approach to management refers to the way in which an organisation works in terms of its purpose and formal structure. The focus is on the planning of work to achieve the organisation's stated aims. It is often confusing when reviewing the literature as 'scientific', 'formal', 'structural' and 'bureaucratic' are all terms used when describing the classical approach to management. Indeed, there are many similarities but it may be useful to examine this approach under two separate headings:

1. Scientific.
2. Bureaucracy.

These two elements are based on the work carried out in the early 1900s by such people as Taylor (1856-1915), Fayol (1949), Brech (1965), Urwick (1952) and Mooney and Reiley (1939). Attempts were made to set out common principles that applied to all organisations. Each protagonist specified a number of principles ranging from fourteen (Fayol) to three (Mooney and Reiley). Those set out by Mooney and Reiley are the ones most often quoted as they can be seen to apply to all types of organisations. The three principles are stated as follows:

1. *The principle of coordination*: the need for people to act together with unity of action, the exercise of authority and the need for discipline.
2. *The scalar principle*: featuring the grading of duties and the process of delegation.
3. *The functional principle*: specialisation and the distinction between different kinds of duties.

Linked to the notion of the scalar principle, Brech indicates a need for job description as an aid to effective organisation and delegation. One element that the evaluative literature does support is that there is little consideration given to the people operating in such conditions. Personality factors, control over working environment and opportunity to be involved in decision making are not considered as important as meeting deadlines in an efficient and effective manner.

Scientific management

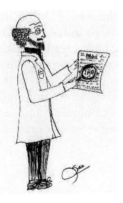

This style of management became evident during the early twentieth century and concentrated on effective and efficient performance of skills in order to increase overall efficiency. Taylor (1856–1915) is often said to be the 'father' of scientific management, and it is he, together with Gilbreth (1868–1924) and Gantt (1861–1919), who continue to influence many organisations today. The foundation of this approach is that there has to be a 'best' working method to achieve the stated goal just as there is a 'best' machine for each job. As you might imagine, the notion of scientific management stems from the achievement of specific objectives through efficiency, standardisation and discipline. It is concerned with finding more efficient methods and procedures for coordination and control of work. Together with this it is about giving the highest possible wages for working in the most efficient and productive way and the development of a true science for each person's work through scientific selection training, the development of the workers, the division of work responsibility between management and the workers, and cooperation with the workers to ensure that work is carried out in the prescribed way.

Taylor's research

At the height of the industrial reorganisation and revolution in the early 1900s, Taylor conducted an experiment at the Bethlehem Steel Corporation, which produced pig iron. He demonstrated that, for each gradient of financial incentive, greater and greater productivity could be achieved. Taylor used one particular man of known limited intelligence in an 'experiment' using a group of seventy-five other workers as the control group. It was shown that, given the right financial incentives of bonuses, four times the amount of productivity could be achieved. The work was divided up into discrete units of activity with little ability for social interaction during the designated work activity. Unfortunately, even after the seventy-five workers were specifically trained to increase their output, only one in eight achieved the maximum output.

> In terms of traditional science, write down what points you think are important about this as an experiment.

You may have thought that it was unethical to use human subjects like this, particular as the experiment used someone who possibly had a learning difficulty. It treated the participants as though they were chemicals or pieces of machinery that could indicate results based on cause and effect. The health and safety issues were not recognised as important at the time. Human life was seen as dispensable. If workers injured themselves or indeed died in trying to earn slightly more money, other workers were just as ready to take over. The experiment never really identified that this type of productivity was sustainable and indeed it did not show that the results were repeatable. The results of the experiments did lead to much criticism at the time and industrial union action by the workers led to a government committee report. Scientific management was said to have offered some useful organisational suggestions and focused on the following:

- efficiency through division of labour
- jobs could be broken down into smaller parts and the most efficient way of completing them could be studied scientifically

- training and development
- motivation through performance pay.

In retrospect, this approach has been criticised because of the management control and the belief that workers were considered units of production at the mercy of capitalism. Despite this, Taylorism still features in many factories today which use this system of 'piece work' and incentive. Indeed, as technology improves, robots are being developed to cope with the repetitive and mundane tasks once performed by people, particularly in the manufacturing industries.

How do you think Taylorism has influenced practice in health care delivery?

Task allocation (Chapter 5) could be thought to be akin to this approach in that nursing care delivery was based on the repetition of tasks related to each patient. It did not recognise the psychological needs of the patient or the nurse delivering the care but concentrated on the specific task to be undertaken.

Do you still see elements of task allocation in nursing practice today?

It can be said that we practise holistic care, but do we really? Many clinical areas are divided into 'areas' or 'ends' and team leaders direct the work for the shift within those areas. Patient care may then be divided into 'bays', individuals or tasks.

Taylor felt that the classical approach to management should be applied to every worker within the organisation in order to maintain and improve efficiency. He also maintained that the relationship between managers and workers would improve, as all concerned would benefit financially. However, Taylor's methods and ideas did not meet with outright approval as it became apparent that the number of people required to raise the efficiency would be fewer as the financial incentives increased. This led to strike action (American Watertown Arsenal 1912) being taken and an investigation of the method by a Committee of the House of Representatives which concluded that 'Scientific management did provide useful techniques' but during 1914 the American Congress banned Taylor's time study methods in its defence industry due to continuing unrest among the workers. Taylorism continued in other areas of industry.

Gilbreth continued Taylor's work but he wanted to refine it further. It was through Gilbreth's work that the notion of 'time and motion' studies came about. In nursing this was particularly noticed during the early 1960s when such tasks as bed-making were examined to see if the number of movements required to make a bed could be reduced. A 'man with a clipboard' started to enter ward areas and examine the way that beds were made, and then return some time later with a new job design of efficient bed making (which is still practised today!). It is interesting to note that the suggested 'new' approach to bed making reflected the old saying 'First the tail and then the head, that's the way to make a bed.' Today community staff also detail each activity in a diary for management and financial data.

Gantt also endeavoured to build on the work of Taylor because he felt that there was a need to humanise the approach. This he did by replacing the 'piece work' scenario with a 'day rate' plus a 20–50 per cent enhancement if targets were met. Gantt wrote:

> The general policy of the past has been to drive. The era of force must give way to that of knowledge; the policy of the future will be to teach and to lead [and] Time is needed to overcome prejudice and change habits. This is a psychological law. Its violation produces failure just as surely as the violation of the laws of physics or chemistry. (Rathe 1961, p. 9)

This indicates that Gantt felt that the worker, as a person, needed to be respected and treated with compassion and dignity, but that he also recognised that the worker was motivated, in the main, by money.

So scientific management did not always look at the individual and therefore did not always work effectively. It assumes that all workers are motivated by money and could therefore be neglected on a personal level. Further, it failed to appreciate how workers would interpret being observed or timed. Together with this the workers' psychological needs were not taken into account. It is not surprising that the notion of scientific management has largely been superseded by more enlightened approaches – or has it?

If Taylor, Gilbreth and Gantt were so outdated in their approaches, why do you imagine that this style of management is still applied in health service provision? Discuss this point with a colleague.

This is rather a rhetorical question depending on the situation. Clearly when there is an emergency it is easier to manage if each person has specific responsibilities in which they are well trained. It can be argued that it leads to more effective and efficient use of labour and is termed 'neo-Taylorism'. We will return to examine this further later in the chapter.

The bureaucratic approach

Encompassed within the classical approach to management is bureaucracy. According to Weber (1947) bureaucracy is the most efficient way of running large organisations. It is documented that Weber (1864–1920), a German sociologist, did not invent the term 'bureaucracy' – that was attributed to de Gourney (1712–59) – but it is Weber who is most often quoted when discussing the main features of this approach which is based on power and authority.

- *power* means the ability to get things done, often by the use of threats or sanctions; whereas
- *authority* means the ability to get things done because of the position that justified you in terms of legitimacy.

Weber studied early societies and identified three types of authority:

1. *Traditional authority* which was based on the notion that the ruler had either the 'God-given' right to rule, as in some dynasties, or that it came to him through descent, e.g. the authority enjoyed by kings.
2. *Charismatic authority* exhibited by people like Hitler and Martin Luther King.
3. *Legal–rational authority* which is based on the formal, written rules, e.g. the prime minister, university deans and principals might all fall into this category.

Weber describes this approach as being formal but also impersonal and rational, very similar to the scientific approach but possibly more calculating and rational in its outlook. Its main characteristics are that within bureaucracy there is hierarchical authority which applies to the organisation of offices and positions. Together with this the tasks of the organisation are allocated as official duties among the various positions and there is an implied, clear-cut division of labour and a high level of specialisation. Uniformity of decisions and actions is achieved through formally established systems of rules and regulations, and an impersonal orientation is expected from officials in their dealings with clients and other officials. Employment by the organisation is based on technical qualifications and may constitute a lifelong career for the officials. Furthermore there is scientific selection, training and development of the workers with the surety that workers will carry out their tasks in a prescribed way. Bureaucracy has strengths in that it demonstrates fairness and gives clarity of responsibilities to workers.

Think about the entry to nurse education and the way in which your career will proceed. Can you see a resemblance of this approach to management?

You will probably have thought of the need to demonstrate that you are able to reach a prescribed academic level in order to commence training. You may also have had to undergo an interview or some form of selection process, and later, to continue practice, there is the need for professional updating. Together with this is the need to satisfy PREP requirements (Chapter 12), to maintain your portfolio (Chapter 4) and to demonstrate your ability to maintain and increase your knowledge, as well as the policies and procedures to be adhered to within clinical practice. You may have thought of many others, all of which can be attributed to the ethos of scientific management and bureaucracy in particular.

Criticisms of bureaucracy

It is said that bureaucracy cannot respond easily to change. Indeed Argyris (1962, 1970) stated that, according to a theory of personality development, as a person matured they would become dissatisfied with the organisational restrictions. Similarly, critics may say that this method of managing an organisation, or part of an organisation, might demonstrate an over-emphasis on rules and procedures, record keeping and paperwork so initiative would be stifled. Officials may develop a dependence on status which could lead to officious behaviour, again leading to a lack of development of maturity. Argyris went on to highlight the frustration that workers would ultimately feel when working in this type of environment and would need to develop coping strategies. The coping strategies he talked about were daydreaming, aggression, regression and projection, restricting production quotas, making errors, slowing down, stealing and sabotage, and demonstrating lack of interest, to name a few. Altogether there would be widespread apathy, not because the workers are lazy but rather because that is the way they are treated, as though they had not got the ability to make decisions; therefore they reacted by living up to expectations (the self-fulfilling prophecy). Argyris then went on to discuss an alternative to bureaucracy which was developed within the Japanese culture. Ouchi (1981) offered a theory that contrasted with the American bureaucracy theory, known as theory Z. Table 7.2 demonstrates the differences between theory A (American) and theory Z (Japanese). It can be seen that, for workers in organisation A, there might be a constant risk of unemployment if they do not 'toe the company line' whereas in organisation Z this would not be the case. Also, because there was consensual decision making, employees did not become disillusioned but enjoyed lifetime employment. However, over the last twenty years it has been noticed that within Japanese industry there has been a willingness to recruit not only from other companies within Japan but also to recruit foreigners in order to shake up the complacent attitude of workers. So while it can be seen that there may be a place for this type of culture as an alternative to bureaucracy, it too has its problems.

As society and organisations recognised the problems with bureaucracy, there was a move towards a more human approach to management. The task was not the only thing to be considered; the people who were doing the various tasks were seen to be workers who should be treated in a more humane way. Thus came the human relations approach to management.

Table 7.2 Characteristics of Theory A and Theory Z organisations

Theory A	Theory Z
Short-term employment	Long-term employment, often for a lifetime
Specialised career paths	Relatively slow process of evaluation and promotion
Individual decision making	Development of company-specific skills, and moderately specialised career path
Individual responsibility	Implicit, informal control mechanisms supported by explicit, formal measures
Frequent appraisal	Participate in decision making by consensus
Explicit, formalised appraisal	Collective decision making but individual ultimate responsibility
Rapid promotion	Broad concern for the welfare of subordinates and
Segmented concern for people	co-workers as a natural part of working relationship, and informal relationships among people

The human relations approach

In the 1920s, management theorists started to pay more attention to the social factors associated with work, i.e. the interrelationship of humans involved within the workplace. As the classical approach studied the structural and formal aspects of work, the human relations approach studied the behavioural or informal aspects of organisational life. The focus was predominantly on workers as people. The main proponent of the human relations approach is Mayo (1880–1949) although it is disputed whether he actually took part in the Hawthorne experiments at the Western Electric Company in America (1924–32). The experiment set out to examine workers in four phases, using initially the scientific approach of control and experimental groups in the research.

Illumination room experiments

The aim of this element of the experiments was to study the relationship between the quality and quantity of light and the various workers' productivity. Findings showed that the level of production was affected by light intensity but lighting was only one factor and that further experiments would be required to see if those factors could be ascertained.

Relay assembly test room

Women who volunteered for this experiment were working a 48-hour week (with no tea breaks) in the relay assembly area and were studied against a control group of the main workforce who had similar physical working conditions. A variety of changes were introduced to see how output was affected. Rest breaks were introduced and then lunch breaks, until later a shorter working day and Saturdays off were tried. All this contributed to increased output and did not appear to decrease even when the women returned to a 48-hour week. The women were then interviewed about the results and indicated that they felt special and involved in the discussions about the changes in their work practices. They also felt that the researcher was friendly towards them, which raised morale; and because they had self-selected with their friends they developed closer interpersonal relationships and so were better able to work as a team.

Interviewing programme

This part of the research involved interviewing employees in confidence to identify their thoughts on their supervisors and working conditions. Initially the interviews were highly structured but after some time they became semi-structured. Employees started to identify the impact of non-work-related topics and were allowed to voice grievances. It was discovered that the workers valued the fact that someone would listen to their concerns and that there was a complex informal structure of the organisation which was much more intricate than the formal structures demonstrated. It was on this basis that personnel work was set up.

Bank wiring observation room

This experiment involved observing how certain social groups exercised control over others in a certain part of the factory. Initially, researchers found that the main group was operating at well below its capacity and those workers were therefore not earning as much as they could have done. Further investigation revealed that the workers were controlling their own outputs as laid down by norms set by the group's informal leaders. This was felt to be because they were afraid of increasing their output as this increase would be continually expected which could lead to redundancies, as fewer people would be required to meet output levels. In order to combat this the group decided, informally, on a level of output that they considered acceptable/reasonable. The rest of the group, through ridicule, negatively sanctioned anyone within the group who worked outside this level.

The Hawthorne studies illustrated new thinking on organisational management, which concentrated on the needs of people as workers. Doing research on people and motivation can often make the participants feel valued and special and therefore affect the outcomes of the research. The Hawthorne studies overall demonstrated four issues:

1. People are motivated by more than just pay and conditions.
2. The need for a sense of belonging and recognition is very important.
3. The attitude to work is shaped by co-workers.
4. The power of the informal organisation must not be underestimated.

But how do these influence health care practice today?

Jot down notes on how each of the four parts of the Hawthorne experiments could be applied to your clinical area.

You may have noted that physical conditions of the work environment are not the only important aspect of enjoying work. Some of the most pleasurable work experiences arise when there is a good team spirit. Interestingly, often the person who is 'doing the off duty' will be aware of who works well with whom and will ensure that people who do not get on well do not work the same shift too often, if at all. Most of us look at the following day's rota to see who we are 'on' with and this knowledge will influence our attitude when arriving at work to commence the shift. However, treating one another with respect leads to a happier workforce. Induction and clinical supervision are important in order to listen to how new recruits and current staff are settling in within the team and to respect any concerns they may have.

Consider how you felt when entering a new clinical area.
• Discuss how you became aware of the informal structure/organisation.
• Jot down how you became accepted by any of the informal groups in the clinical area.
• If that was not your experience, jot down the difficulty you had if you felt you remained an 'outsider'.

Students often remark that they feel 'outsiders' when entering a new clinical area, most particularly when placed in departments. This can be said to reflect the findings of the Hawthorne experiments, and the interviewing programme in particular, where it is demonstrated that the social grouping appears to exercise a great deal of influence over the notion of 'belonging'. Many private hospitals have taken on board the findings of the Hawthorne studies in their approach to the development of their hospitals. The wards are carpeted, there are televisions and telephones in the rooms, and the whole ambience of their units is one of quiet, well-lit calm. There are perhaps fewer nurses on duty but the work still gets completed. All staff are cared for, often receiving free meals on duty and being able to access private medical care for themselves and their family either as part of their employment rights or at a reduced rate. All these elements demonstrate a caring employer taking a human relations approach to management.

The systems approach

While the classical approach is often thought to be an approach that does not consider people, only the organisation, the human relations approach considers people but does not necessarily consider the organisation. By contrast the systems approach encourages managers to view the organisation both as a whole and also as part of a wider environment. Exponents of the approach include von Bertalanffy (1951), Walker and Guest (1952), Sayles (1958), Blauner (1964), Miller and Rice (1967) and Woodward (1980). The common consensus is that organisations have similar features to a socio-technical system which links technical aspects of the job with the social system in which they fit.

During the 1950s Walker and Guest (1952) studied people who worked on a production line within a car assembly plant. They were attempting to see how satisfied the workers were with their working terms and conditions. Interestingly, they were satisfied with pay, working conditions and quality of supervision but very dissatisfied with the actual work they were doing. There were six main factors responsible for this dissatisfaction:

1. Mechanical pacing over which they had no control.
2. Repetitive work.
3. Low level of skill required.
4. Involvement with only a small part of the overall process.
5. Limited social interaction with colleagues.
6. No control over the methods or tools used to do the job.

In the light of this, alternative approaches to work practices were developed.

Job rotation

Here workers move around in a systematic way from one area to another in order to improve interest and motivation. Increasingly this can be seen to be being implemented within nursing and midwifery whereby newly qualified staff are offered rotational contracts on qualification so that they spend six months or so in a variety of settings (often three) before specialising in one particular area. At ward level, staff may be encouraged to experience periods of night duty on a rotational basis. Again this is being built into contracts but

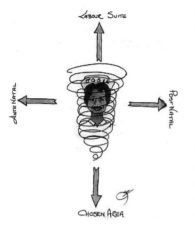

assumes that there will be an increase in motivation and interest, while there would be a decrease in the 'them and us' feeling as each set of staff will understand the pressures and stresses of each other's workload.

Job enlargement

This is often called *horizontal job loading* because it links to the expansion of the worker's role by including tasks traditionally performed by other workers. The rationale behind this is that by increasing the complexity of the role there would be renewed interest and greater motivation, thus reducing boredom. Within the delivery of health care we know that nurses and midwives are being trained to take on many roles that, traditionally, used to belong to junior doctors.

Can you name some of them?

You may have considered venepuncture, giving IV drugs, prescribing (but limited to a specific range of drugs and dressings), suturing and referral to other services, to name a few. However, job enlargement does not really live up to expectations as nurses and midwives often do not see this as enriching their jobs – only making them larger and more complex but with very little time or income to support their extra duties.

Job enrichment

Due to the adverse reactions to job enlargement and job rotation, this notion was proposed. Job enrichment is based on Hertzberg's (1966) theory whereby he says that people are motivated towards what makes them feel good. The work of nurses, midwives and health visitors can be based on this, in that the five areas that Hertzberg identifies are being addressed with professional practice:

1. *Accountability*: Nurses, midwives and health visitors are held responsible for their own practice and performance (UKCC 1992).

2. *Achievement*: Nurses, midwives and health visitors should feel that they are doing something of worth. This is the very nature of this type of work.

3. *Feedback*: Nurses, midwives and health visitors should receive feedback related to their performance. Such activities as annual performance review are becoming commonplace. While they may be seen as threaten-

ing in the first instance, they can be used to identify training and development needs and so aid effective planning.

4. *Work pace*: At times there appears to be little possibility for nurses, midwives and health visitors to set their own pace of work as it often depends on the demands of the patients/clients of the day.

5. *Control over resources*: While this element may be limited within health care provision it can be seen that the 'G' grade nurses now do hold a budget allocated to the clinical area of work.

The contingency approach

During the 1950s writers began to consider alternatives to classical and human relations approaches to the management of organisations. They started to develop a structure based on 'it all depends', recognising that those management approaches might change within given situations. So it is about trying to achieve some degree of fit between the tasks, the people performing the tasks and the environment in which the tasks are to be undertaken. It will be the prevailing circumstances that dictate the best way of achieving the goal for that situation.

Huczynski and Buchanan (1991) state:

> It is worthwhile stressing that whilst writers talk about contingency theory, it is nothing of the sort. It is more correct to consider it as a way of thinking rather than a set of interrelated causal elements which might be said to constitute a theory. (Huczynski and Buchanan 1991, p. 454)

Broadly speaking, the activities within an organisation can be classed as follows:

- *steady state*: i.e. routine activities
- *policy making*: identifying goals, setting standards and allocating resources
- *innovation*: anything that changes the company research and development departments
- *breakdown*: occurring when dealing with crisis and emergency situations.

There is debate related to whether the size of the company, its technology or overall mission have a part to play in the management approach applied and which, in turn, rely on the informal organisation, personalities and teamwork.

Porter *et al.* (1975) suggested that the size of an organisation is linked to its behaviour. Their work revealed that in the larger units there was a clear negative correlation between job satisfaction, absenteeism and staff turnover. However, Child (1975) found that the larger the company, the greater the relationship between bureaucracy and superior performance. Other writers – Woodward (1980), Perrow (1970), Burns and Stalker (1966), Lawrence and

Lorsch (1969) – have indicated that the contingency approach appears to provide further insight into the relationship between organisational structure and the demands of the environment.

Overall the contingency approach depends on the situation in which the manager is operating. It rejects the notion that there is one best method of management but assumes that the organisation is flexible and can adapt to any given situation.

> Perhaps you can think of times when you use the contingency approach when managing your time and finances.

You might have thought about how you manage time in order to achieve all you need to for successful completion of the course. Do you ever get to the stage where you are trying to work out what not to do in order that you can present an assignment on time? Or is there too much month left at the end of the money? Whatever the situation, you will have to draw up some kind of contingency plan in order to achieve your aims.

Management by objectives

Drucker (1989) described management by objectives (MBO) as a collection of activities designed to aid workers in meeting the goals or mission of the organisation. It involves planning, organisation, direction and control of all the activities within the workplace. The underlying basis of the system is as follows:

- setting objectives and targets
- participation by individual managers in agreeing unit objectives and criteria of performance
- reviewing and appraising results.

Mullins (2000) describes the cycle of MBO interrelated activities (Figure 7.2) wherein the cyclical nature of the system is depicted. This might indicate that in order to be fully effective the objectives also need to be linked to a system that allows career progression or other awards to be the driving force behind the work ethic. The agreement of targets is not imposed but democratically decided through discussion between managers and their subordinates so that, provided that the overall goal/mission is achieved, the work will continue at the pace and direction determined, i.e. a participative style of management practice. We can see in nursing, midwifery and health visiting an increasing emphasis being put on annual individual performance review (IPR) which, though not linked to career progression directly, does place emphasis on the professionals identifying their objectives for the year. Together with this is the Post-Registration Education Project (PREP) (UKCC 1998) which requires that all professionals demonstrate that they have made attempts to maintain their professional knowledge through reading, taking courses or investigating the work practices of others in order to enhance care provision. These activities take time to plan, put into practice and evaluate their effectiveness (which are all elements of MBO) if they are to succeed.

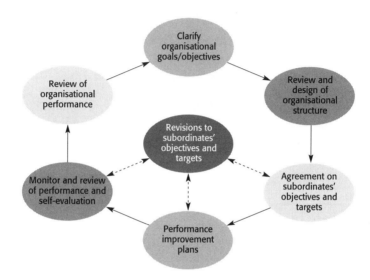

Figure 7.2 The cycle of MBO activities

In order to be really successful an MBO approach requires commitment and active support from management in the form of setting key goals or targets. As with any democratic situation, time is required for discussion in order to ascertain the needs or requirements of others. Similarly, time is required to evaluate their effectiveness through measurement against the set standards. Together with this is the need for genuine participation. It is obvious that if, through IPR, areas of personal development need are identified, there must be time set aside in order that those needs are met. If this is not the case, then IPR becomes a sterile activity, a paper exercise. In relation to nursing, midwifery and health visiting, meeting (PREP) requirements must not become a chore – rather, it must be seen as an activity that enhances care delivery and as such is an enjoyable activity.

So MBO is a potentially attractive system which provides the opportunity for staff to accept responsibility for practice and make greater contributions within the workplace. Mullins (2000) lists the following ten advantages:

1. Concentrates attention on main areas where it is important for the organisation to be effective.
2. Identifies problem areas in progress towards achievement of objectives.
3. Improves management control information and performance standards.
4. Leads to a sound organisational structure, clarifies responsibilities, and aids delegation and coordination.
5. Identifies where changes are needed and seeks continual improvement in results.
6. Aids management succession planning.
7. Identifies training needs, and provides an environment that encourages personal growth and self-discipline.
8. Improves appraisal systems, and provides more equitable procedure for determining rewards and promotion plans.
9. Improves communications and interpersonal relationships.
10. Encourages motivation to improve individual performance.

As with all management approaches, MBO is subject to a number of criticisms and potential limitations but it has been likened to the 'modern' form of scientific management in that there will still be a senior management team, job descriptions, policies, procedures, roles and responsibilities. It is, however, noticeable that in some instances the formation of 'objective statements' and targets might be difficult to quantify or measure in precise terms, so it may be that at this point there will be a need to address the issue from another perspective. Management over control may also equate to the MBO approach.

Conclusion

This chapter has attempted to link a variety of management theories to the practice of nursing, midwifery and health visiting. It can be seen that no one style of management approach is effective in all situations. However, within the National Health Service the overall structure appears to be one of a scientific nature with sets of rules, regulations and policies governing the functions of the organisation throughout. Some areas, however, are less bureaucratic than others but there appears to be a 'drive' towards more scientific management as the link with accountability grows stronger, e.g. audits, care pathways. On the other hand, the value of the human relations approach is still recognised in the health service, for example aesthetically pleasing architectural plans for general hospitals with dining restaurants that are less like canteens and more based on social grouping interests.

Summary of key points

During this chapter we have examined a variety of management theories and how they might, individually, be applied to situations within the health care arena. In particular:

- **Importance of management theory:** In order to function effectively it is vital that management theory is understood, for with understanding will come increased efficiency and effectiveness in achieving the purpose of the organisation.

- **Basic components of an organisation:** Within any organisation there is a structure or hierarchy, each layer having its own roles and responsibilities. Most of us spend our working lives trying to reach the next 'rung' on this organisational ladder.

- **The formal and informal organisation:** Described some of the differences between these two elements that coexist within any organisation and will be addressed again in Chapter 8.

- **The classical approach to management:** Discussed the features that, while being first identified in the early nineteenth century, are still apparent within organisational structure today in order to maintain productivity. Whether within a factory or the NHS, productivity is still a major driving force.

- **The human relations approach:** Takes an alternative view to the classical approach in that it attempts to recognise people working within the organisation, demonstrating the need for a 'human' approach in relation to team working.

- **The systems approach:** Here we examined work practices that are reflected today throughout the NHS in such practices as job rotation, enlargement and enrichment – all practices that, it is suggested, help with job satisfaction and so enhance staff retention through maintaining interest.

- **The contingency approach:** Depends on the situation in which a manager is operating in much the same way as we manage our own time and finances outside the employment environment.

- **Management by objectives:** Looks at a way in which we can all be involved in assisting the organisation to meet its aims and outcomes.

References

Argyris C (1962) *Interpersonal competence and organizational effectiveness*, Richard D. Irwin

Argyris C (1970) *Personality and Organizational Freedom between Systems and the Individual*, Harper and Row

Atkinson J (1984) Manpower strategies for flexible organisations, *Personnel Management*, August, 28–31

Blauner R (1964) *Alienation & Freedom*, University of Chicago Press

Brech E F L (1965) *Organisations: The Framework of Management* (2nd edn) Longman

Broome A (1998) *Managing Change*, (2nd edn) Macmillan

Burns T and Stalker G M (1966) *The Management of Innovation*, Tavistock Publications

Burns T and Stalker G M (1994) *The Management of Innovation*, (rev. edn) Oxford University Press

Child J (1975) Organisation: *A Guide to Problems and Practice* (2nd edn) Paul Chapman

Clark J and Copcutt L (1997) *Management for Nurses and Health Care Professionals*, Churchill Livingstone

Department of Health (1999) *Report of the NHS Taskforce on Staff Involvement*, The Stationery Office

Department of Health (Peach Report) (1999) *Making a Difference*, The Stationery Office

Drucker P F (1989) *The Practice of Management*, Heinemann Professional

Fayol H (1949) *General and Industrial Management*, Pitman

Gray J L and Starke F A (1984) *Organizational Behaviour: Concepts and Applications* (3rd edn) Charles E Merrill

Handy C (1985) *Understanding Organisations*, Penguin

Handy C (1989) *The Age of Unreason*, Business Books

Hertzberg F (1966) *Work and the Nature of Man*, Staples Press

Huczynski A and Buchanan D (1991) *Organizational Behaviour: An Introductory Text* (2nd edn) Prentice Hall

Lawrence P R and Lorsch J W (1969) *Organisation and Enviroment*, Irwin

Lysons K (1997) Organisational Analysis, supplement to *The British Journal of Administrative Management*, 18, March/April

Macleod Nicol N and Walker S (1991) *Basic Management for Staff Nurses*, Chapman & Hall

Miller E J and Rice A K (1967) *Systems of Organisations*, Tavistock Publications

Miner J B (1980) *Theories of Organisational Behaviour*, Dryden Press

Mooney J D and Reiley A C (1939) *The Principles of Organization*, Harper and Bros., revised by Mooney J D (1947) Harper and Row

Mullins L J (2000) *Management and Organisational Behaviour* (5th edn) Pitman

Northcott N (1999) Effective staff, *Nursing Times Learning Curve* 3(8), 10

Ouchi W (1981) *Theory Z: How American Business Can Meet the Japanese Challenge*, Addison Wesley

Ouchi W G and Haeger A M (1978) Type Z organisations: stability in the midst of mobility, *Academy of Management Review*, April, 303

Pearcey P (2000) Role perceptions of auxiliary nurses: an exploratory study, *NT Research* 5(1), 55–63

Perrow C (1970) *Organisational Analysis: A Sociological View*, Tavistock Publications

Porter L W, Lawler C H and Hackman J R (1975) *Behavior in Organisations*, McGraw-Hill

Rathe A W (1961) *Gnatt on Management*, American Management Association

Sayles L R (1958) *Behaviour of Industrial Work Groups*, Wiley

Taylor F W (1947) *Scientific Management*, Harper and Row

UKCC (1992) *Code of Professional Practice*, UKCC

UKCC (1998) *Post Registration Education and Training*, UKCC

UKCC (1999) *Fitness for Practice*, UKCC

Urwick L (1952) *Notes on the Theory of Organisations*, American Management Association

von Bertalanffy L (1951) Problems of general systems theory: a new approach to the unity of science, *Human Biology*, **23**(4), December 1951

Walker C R and Guest R H (1952) *The Men on the Assembly Line*, Harvard University Press

Weber M (1947) *The Theory of Social and Economic Organisations*, Collier Macmillan

Woodward J (1980) *Industrial Organisations: Theory & Practice* (2nd edn) Oxford University Press

Further reading

Argyris C (1960) *Understanding Organizational Behaviour*, Tavistock Publications

Argyris C (1964) *Integrating the Individual and the Organization*, Wiley

Armstrong M (1990) *Management Processes and Functions*, Institute of Personnel Management

DuGay P (2000) *In Praise of Bureaucracy*, Sage

Faulkner A (1985) *Nursing – A Creative Approach*, Baillière Tindall

Gantt H (1919) *Organising for Work*, Harcourt, Brace and Hove

Gilbreth F B (1908) *Field System*, Myron C Clarke Publishing

Gilbreth F B and Gilbreth L (1916) *Fatigue Study*, Sturgis & Walton

Gross R D (1987) *Psychology: The Science of Mind and Behaviour*, Hodder & Stoughton

Iles V (1997) *Really Managing Health Care*, Open University Press

Makin P, Cooper C and Cox C (1989) *Managing People at Work*, The British Psychological Society and Routledge

McGhie A (1986) *Psychology as Applied to Nursing*, (8th edn) Churchill Livingstone

McKenna E (1994) *Business Psychology & Organisational Behaviour: A Students' Handbook*, Lawrence Erlbaum Associates

Millar B and Burnard P (1994) *Critical Care Nursing*, Baillière Tindall

Quinn F M (1995) *The Principles and Practice of Nurse Education*, (3rd edn) Chapman & Hall

Sperling A (1957) *Psychology Made Simple*, W H Allen

Sullivan E J and Decker P J (1997) *Effective Leadership and Management in Nursing*, (4th edn) Addison-Wesley

Weber A L (1992) *Social Psychology*, Harper Perennial

Williams H (1994) *The Essence of Managing People*, Prentice Hall

8

Managing change

By the end of this chapter you will have had the opportunity to:

- examine the nature of change
- review your knowledge of change theory
- describe the change process
- identify change within yourself
- discuss change within the team
- examine organisational change
- discuss the skills required to become a successful change agent
- develop a strategy for managing change within yourself, the team and the organisation incorporating:
  - forces for and against change
  - key players
  - resources
  - time scale
- discuss ways to handle resistance to change.

Introduction

The final chapter in this part attempts to draw together elements of team working to effect change. The previous chapters within this part have examined organising care (Chapter 5), leadership (Chapter 6) theoretical considerations (Chapter 7) and now we will look at managing change.

This chapter will examine change theory, linking it to you, the team and the organisation by examining the nature of change, the change process and the skills required to become a successful change agent. It will also examine some of the strategies that could be incorporated in effectively managing change by analysing sources of resistance to change and approaches that may be adopted in order to reduce the resistance. Florence Nightingale (1873;

cited in van der Peet 1995) recognised the need for change when she talked about it in relation to social improvement. Equally her ideas could be applied to present-day care delivery in order to enhance the patient/client experience because every time we learn something new we will have to consider whether change is appropriate. Change is inevitable, even if it is not always welcome. Change is all around us and evolutionary theory teaches us that 'all organisms must adapt with their environment or die' (Iles 1997) so it is necessary to understand the concept of change and the effective management of it.

The nature of change

Huczynski and Buchanan (1991) highlight that rapid change is commonplace. They note that complexity, disorganisation and frustration are all natural aspects of our daily lives. The nature of change is also hard to study as it is difficult to stand back from a routine process in which one is constantly involved and look at it objectively.

> Change is not a single process or group of processes: It ... does not exist at all. It is an ideal, a story made by everyone who is experiencing discontinuity. Viewed as a cause of events, by others as a consequence, it can be the disease, diagnosis and the cure. (Clarke and Copcutt 1997)

So we may view change differently and it will affect us at home, at work and at leisure in different ways. It is also important to realise that it

- can cause anxiety and uncertainty
- is not often welcomed
- is inevitable
- may be imposed.

Indeed, change occurs without us realising at times and is therefore invisible. As nurses, midwives and health visitors we need to recognise the impact and implications of change within our professional work, which may be brought about by the political, economic or social systems affecting health care. It is also an important element for the patients and clients we care for as they face change and, for some, rapid change in their health status. Helping others through change means that we should have some understanding of the impact and effect on all concerned.

Think of a recent change that has been brought into a clinical area such as new rotas, care pathways or the introduction of new clinical guidelines. Write down some of the staff's feelings that they may have mentioned to you. Do these fit in with this view of uncertainty and concern?

Some may feel resigned, others may be excited and others may be angry or annoyed. Others may attempt to ignore the proposed change but, in general, the concern for the uncertainty is felt. This may be because of the unknown *personal* effect as well as how it will impact professionally.

The need for change

'Change for change's sake' is a phrase sometimes uttered when people are feeling overwhelmed by imposed newness. However, it has to be said that all change is not necessary. Some change is even difficult to evaluate years after it has occurred. Project 2000 (P2K) was a dramatic change to

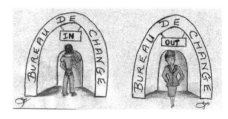

our professional training and education. There has been much resistance and difficulty in accepting that nursing can have an acknowledged powerbase worthy of a pre-registration higher educational award. However, this type of training should not have jeopardised the practical skills and competencies required for registered practice. Indeed health visiting and district nursing went into higher education many decades previously with little concern.

Discuss with a few staff in different clinical areas who were P2K trained and non-P2K trained whether they regretted or were pleased with their own training. What advantages and disadvantages do they highlight?

Whether P2K was the right change is still a matter of debate but that change was seen as necessary in order to help students to think critically about holistic care. This is particularly pertinent now in the light of clinical governance today. Ritualistic practice is a risk and, as risks lead to litigation, it can be expensive when Trusts are deemed liable.

Rogers and Shoemaker (1971) identified seven criteria that are useful in evaluating the success of innovative practice for the future:

1. *Relative advantage*: unless there is relative advantage in change over the *status quo*, there is likely to be no impetus for change.
2. *Compatibility*: this concerns the proposed change 'fitting' with existing philosophy and values.
3. *Communicability*: this attribute concerns the ease with which the change can be understood. Communicability is linked both to features of change and to facets of the communicator.

4. *Simplicity*: concerns the ease or difficulty in use of innovation. Difficulties may arise in the understanding of changes, or in their implementation.

5. *Trialability*: concerns the possibility of 'piloting' the innovation on either a small or large scale. A successful trial can lead to a 'ripple' effect whereby change in one group can influence the adoption of change by others.

6. *Observability*: this attribute is self-explanatory in that the benefits must be seen to be accepted.

7. *Relevance*: for meaningful change to take place it must be seen to be relevant.

> Make notes on these points in the light of any new curriculum changes in your professional area that you know about, e.g. fitness for practice (UKCC 1999) recommendations for one year Common Foundation and two years branch specific, or it could be nurse prescribing or changing childbirth recommendations.

Building on this work, Upton and Brooks (1995) identify that for *successful change* to occur there should be a combination of the following:

- dissatisfaction with the present situation
- a vision of a more desirable future
- a knowledge of the first steps to take in moving to that future.

Identify how you think these three areas related to those changes above. These three issues really need to be *greater* than the resistance to or the cost of that change. So before any change is contemplated, there needs to be an exercise that identifies the need for change and the forces that may influence the success or failure of that change (Figure 8.1). This is referred to as a *force field analysis* (Chapter 2) in which a variety of factors are identified, all of which are working either for or against the change.

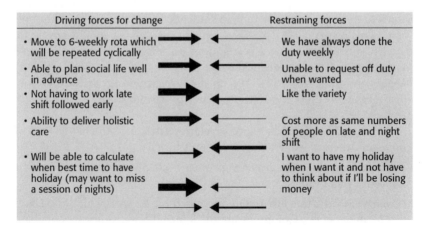

Figure 8.1 Force field analysis for change in method of devising off-duty rosters

- Identify a change you would like to make in your personal life (e.g. losing weight; writing better assignments, stopping smoking).
- List the restraining forces keeping you from making this change.
- List the driving forces that make you want to change.
- Determine how you might be able to change the *status quo* and make the change possible.

You can see from the example in Figure 8.1 that some of the forces for change are stronger than those against. This can be an indication of the need for, and possible success of, the proposed change. It is quite a useful exercise to undertake when making an important decision in your life. Sometimes you will hear people talking about listing the 'pros' and 'cons' of a situation – this is part of force field analysis but you also have to measure the strength of each factor and decide whether it is a driving or restraining force, in order to see where there is possibility for change and in what direction.

The change process

Does change occur naturally or is it planned? It can happen in both ways. Tappen (1995) feels that change *should* occur as a planned event rather than by accident or drift. It is planned change that requires deliberate acts and the application of knowledge and skills by a leader or change agent. Indeed, as health care workers you will often act in this role. Sometimes you will come to work and not have the usual staff and will need to think of doing things differently to help the team to get on with the work, and you will be responsible for this change. The change of staff may not be planned but your actions to delegate and lead the team will involve planned change.

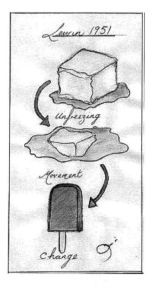

As you can imagine, there are many theories relating to the change process. Many appear to identify elements from the theory first expounded by Lewin (1951) in which he suggests three phases of the change process. These phases relate to:

1. *Unfreezing*: this is the stage to reduce the forces that maintain the status quo. This is where recognition for change and improvement occur
2. *Movement (or change)*: this stage involves taking on board new attitudes or behaviours towards implementing the new change.

3. *Re-freezing*: this is where change is stabilised at a new level and seen as accepted within policies, structures and norm values.

Each of these stages may incorporate certain elements that reflect the particular stage (Table 8.1). From a planning point of view, the ease and speed of change will be affected by recognition of these relevant elements and planned change will be a preferred option. However, change may not run smoothly because there are often constraints holding on to the *status quo*.

Table 8.1 Stages of change and responsibilities of the change agent

Stage 1 – Unfreezing

1. Triggers for change
2. Challenge to *status quo*
3. New power
4. Involvement of outsiders

Do not proceed to Step 2 until the *status quo* has been disrupted, and others perceive the need for change.

Step 2 – Movement (or change)

1. Planned action
2. Enhancing or reducing status
3. Identification of supporters and resisters

Stage 3 – Re-freezing

1. Adaptation
2. New meanings to individuals requiring support

From Lewin (1951)

Change within yourself

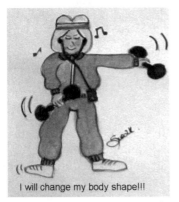
I will change my body shape!!!

You may have heard the phrase 'change incurs opportunities': this is certainly true as you go through your education and training. You will have an opportunity to change the way you see or do things; and you will gradually change the way you act with patients and their relatives due to your increased knowledge. The changes you make within yourself will be influenced by various things – the environment, the peer group you are in and the team, to name a few. 'No pain, no gain' is a phrase that indi-

cates that change is often a painful experience due to the pressures, dissonance or mismatch that it causes. You may hear change being referred to as
internal or external change. Internal change is when, as you might imagine,
something changes within yourself but over which you may have no influence, such as maturity or an experience. External change relates to the
environment, e.g. changing clinical areas, taking on a new training course,
changing political power in government. Looking over your past life seems
to be a way in which you can identify the changes you have already coped
with. This may assist you in the future for, by reflecting on the strategies you
used to cope, you will be able to cope more effectively in later life.

Draw a 'peak and trough' map of your life, highlighting the positive and negative
changes you have coped with.

Your life map might resemble that in Figure 8.2 or it may be rather more
complicated, but broadly there will be three main areas – education, employment, and relationships. How you draw this map will be entirely up to you
but, however you do it, you will get an idea of all the changes you have coped
with already. You may not always notice the change in yourself but others
may remark on it and this gives you an opportunity to reflect on the impact
of change on your life. Indeed, some positive and negative changes are perceived differently by different people.

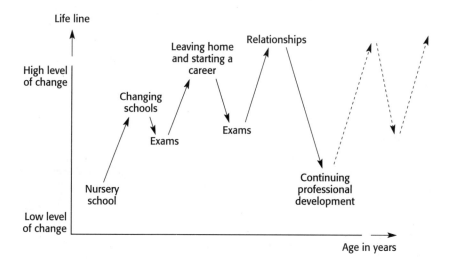

Figure 8.2 Life map

How do you think you have changed since you entered higher education?

- You might even ask a relative or friend (who is not undertaking this course) if they think you have changed.
- You could also consider what part this course has played in your change.

You may have thought about being in charge of your own life, living independently, learning how to manage study with family life and responsibilities. Whatever it is, something will have had to change in order for you to cope with the demands of the course. A student explained that her parents thought that she was changing – they thought she was becoming hard and dispassionate in the way she treated people. It worried her until she thought it through. It occurred to her, on reflection, that before she began nursing she had not been exposed to some of the illnesses and problems that her patients/clients seemed to accept as 'being normal'. On reviewing her feelings and emotions, she developed an understanding of the issues and how different people respond in different ways. By going through this exercise she developed coping and learning strategies which in turn changed her ideas and values about the way things are in other people's lives, and allowed her to recognise how she had to come to terms with the reality of these new situations. This may then have appeared to others that she had become hardened to the situation whereas she was only coping in a way that suited her.

During 1999 the Department of Health released a document called *Making a Difference* (Chapter 12) which calls for nurses, midwives and health visitors to update their practice and underpinning knowledge throughout their careers. In much the same way PREP (UKCC 1999) (Chapter 12) advocates the need to keep up to date in terms of your knowledge which is underpinning your practice. By examining your ability to change you will then become more effective as a team member and will learn to cope with change more effectively.

Change within the team

It could be said that the NHS introduces many changes simultaneously. Some of the changes are larger and are brought about more quickly than others, and others are brought in more slowly. Some of the topical changes may be:

- clinical supervision
- skill mix
- patient-focused care
- nurse and midwifery educational changes

- local pay and conditions
- day surgery
- team midwifery
- nurse prescribing
- introduction of critical care pathways
- clinical governance.

The complexity of change is therefore problematic. This can be overwhelming, having so much change thrust upon us. Some people within the team seem to be able to cope with all these challenges to the *status quo* while others really find they can do no more than turn up for work, hoping the change will pass over without them.

Change within the organisation

Peters and Waterman (1995) noted in their 'excellence literature' that 'excellent firms don't believe in excellence – only in constant improvement and constant change'. This refers to the point that as the environment changes, the excellence of last year is not always the excellence of this year or next year. Therefore change is necessary to keep up with the environment or external environment:

> All organisations are, to a greater or lesser extent, in a perpetual state of change. To survive and thrive ... they must innovate, develop, expand, reorganise, introduce new technology and change working methods and practices. (Armstrong 1990)

However, organisational change creates an impact on the following:

- people
- information
- tasks
- structures
- rewards

whether those organisations are large or small. If you think about the introduction of information technology in health care, you will recognise the impact on *people* to learn new skills. *Information* needs have now changed, particularly in the light of commissioning, clinical governance and National Service Frameworks; tasks such as collating and inputting information into a database have taken on new importance. New *structures* such as information departments have been developed and *recognition and rewards* may be given to those who are familiar or proficient in dealing with information technology tasks. For example, the nurse who is able to access the Internet to gather information for practice may be more highly regarded than one who cannot.

Organisational change creates uncertainty as to what the future holds, and as a consequence this can lead to feelings of insecurity for everyone. However, Burke (1982) suggested that it was not the thought of change as such that created resistance to change but the sense of personal loss which accompanies the change that may cause problems. Change within an organisation is complex. Proposed change could begin with the organisation defining its business and purpose again via a 'mission statement'. The best way to meet the aims of the organisation has to be considered. Invariably there are demands from the environment, which interact with the formal and informal structures of the organisation in order to effect that change. In order to be certain of reaching the organisational goal it is therefore necessary to be aware of change theory and the nature of the change. This, then, recognises the need for effective planning in order to cause the least amount of stress and dissonance in the workforce. New clinical units, colleges of nursing and midwifery that moved into higher education and even new primary care groups and Trusts have all had to put these principles into practice.

Nurses, midwives and health visitors as change agents

Health care professionals are now at a point where they are taking on new roles and skills and playing a main part in commissioning, clinical governance and consultancy. This means that they will be actively involved in change to help the health service run more effectively and efficiently. Nurses, midwives and health visitors have also become more politically aware due to the changing educational input and experience. Despite having had many changes imposed on them in the past, they may be more likely to look for opportunities for changing the *status quo*. They are also possibly in a better position to take a more predominant role in initiating changes for the better, rather than accepting imposed changes. Even newly qualified staff will be expected to take on board personal continuous improvement through clinical supervision and reflective practice right from their first post. This means that there is a need to understand the role of an 'agent of change'.

Change agent skills

In order to become an effective change agent it is necessary to be:

- a problem seeker
- a problem solver
- an innovator
- a leader.

This may seem a tall order in professional practice but this is visible through-out many clinical areas without people realising the roles they play.

One occasion that we remember is when a member of the night staff had to go home at 10.30 p.m. due to a family emergency. The 'F' grade brought us all together to communicate the problem and redistributed the evening work of primary nursing care of the patients in the surgical unit. Most of the patients had been settled but we all lent a hand to complete the work and effect a 'lights out' situation. Highly dependent patients recently back from surgery were prioritised and eventually all patients were settled by 11.30 p.m. During this time the 'F' grade contacted a senior nurse, who knew the patients and was coming on duty the next morning, to communicate the problem. This member of staff volunteered various options:

- to come on duty an hour earlier at 7.00 a.m. to help with the morning work
- to bring an extra agency nurse on day shift to cover the morning workload not covered by the night staff
- to bring an agency nurse in as soon as possible to replace the 'lost' member of staff.

Considering all options and the time taken to transfer information to new staff, it was agreed that the senior member would come in at 7.00 a.m. to help with the workload. Problem solving meant that the night staff were less stressed as they knew they had cover at the busiest time in the morning, they knew the staff member coming on duty, the staff member knew the patients and they were able to manage the boundary between night and day shift. This meant that the night staff were able to give good patient care as they themselves were less stressed. The nurse who came in early was able to leave work early on a shift to suit her before her annual leave, so enabling her to get an early flight for her holiday. In resolving this problem, patients, night staff, day staff and the staff with the emergency achieved a win–win situation. While this illustrates effective problem solving, the changes were not permanent and the effect was brought about by minimal staff changes.

Planning and managing effective change

Planning and managing change depends on whether it is seen as short-, medium- or long-term. The example above relates to a short-term problem and faces us daily at work. The hardest change to effect is one that is long-term.

Write down some examples of a long-term change that you know about.

Long-term issues often relate to changes in working practices, changing mindsets, changing education/training issues. When Jill was involved in child protection training, the need to address multi-agency working was underpinned by the various attitudes to child care and discipline. Police members were mainly concerned with adults crossing the line of the law. Teachers and nursery staff were often concerned with 'fitting with a certain establishment's expectations', social workers were concerned with 'at risk' families, nurses were concerned with medical issues, and health visitors were concerned with growth and development in the broadest sense. Age, ethnicity and gender also complicated the picture of expectations. All of these are right for protecting children, but these expectations need to be brought together and understood in order to help families in multi-agency working. Planned training along these lines involved a long-term aim to bring the various cultures of professionals together.

Gray (1985) stated:

> Planned change is conscious and deliberate, and some attention is given to the way in which it is brought about. It is essentially a political activity; such change depends much on the mood of the times and the skills and resources of the innovators. ... There is no means of distinguishing the one from the other since the natural concept of 'planning change' may be one of natural social changes that are taking place. (Gray 1985, p. 72)

In order to manage change there are six main stages that need to be considered, which are linked to problem solving and leadership:

1. Diagnosing the present situation.
2. Identifying the scope and extent of the change required.
3. Analysing the gap and the transition required to fill that gap.
4. Creating a vision for the future.
5. Handling resistance.
6. Stabilising the new situation.

Knowledge and experience will help in the change process to ensure success. Once an obvious change needs to be made, some planned action needs to be thought through. Teasdale (1992) identifies some strategies for managing people through change within an area of work:

1. Create ownership and involvement.
2. Create a positive environment for change.
3. Work with staff to develop a plan.
4. Communicate the changes.
5. Anticipate conflicts and resistance.

Sometimes change activity will require steering groups or working parties and the structure of these need to be thought through carefully. *Key people* or *stakeholders* will be required. It may be useful to bring on board those people who will struggle with the change process so that their views and opinions may be heard at an earlier stage. There will need to be others who are keen on action and will move a project forward. However, the power and influence within those groups should also be analysed in order to evaluate how it may function.

Chinn (1988) identified three key ways of managing change:

1. *Empirical – rational (selling)*: This is based on the idea that people are rational and will behave according to rational self-interest. It is therefore expected that people will change if they see justification and benefit from it.
2. *Normative – re-educative*: This is based on the assumption that people will act according to the attitudes and values of their norm reference group.
3. *Power coercive (telling)*: This is based on the assumption that the least powerful should comply under the leadership of the most powerful. Conflict is a common feature.

The first two strategies for change can show that, through good communication and group work, change becomes more acceptable, and this was how the child protection change was managed. The third strategy is more problematical, and power within groups and working parties needs to be monitored. Power is a complex concept when dealing with change. Handy (1985) identified five sources of power that could influence the task of any group or working party:

1. *Physical*: strength; physical force; coercion.
2. *Resource*: control of resources:
   ● psychological – status
   ● physical – money and materials
3. *Position*: legitimate; rules and procedures.

4. *Expert*: increased knowledge over others.
5. *Personal*: charisma.

Practitioners need to be aware of how these sources of power can influence change positively or negatively in the control of others. These who feel disempowered invariably resist change.

Ways to handle resistance to change

Table 8.2 Ten emotional phases of the change process

Equilibrium	Noted by high energy and emotional and intellectual balance. Personal and professional goals are synchronised.
Denial	Practitioner denies reality of the change. Negative changes occur in physical, cognitive and emotional functioning.
Anger	Energy is manifested by rage, envy and resentment.
Bargaining	In an attempt to eliminate the change, energy is used in bargaining.
Chaos	Noted by diffused energy, feelings of powerlessness, insecurity and loss of identify.
Depression	Defence mechanisms are no longer operable. Self-pity is in evidence.
Resignation	Change accepted passively but without enthusiasm.
Openness	Some willingness to accept new roles or assignments that have resulted from the change.
Readiness	Wilful expenditure of energy to explore new event. Physical, cognitive and emotional elements involved.
Re-emergence	Practitioner again feels empowered and begins initiating projects and ideas.

It is natural that changes cause discomfort. Indeed, Table 8.2 suggests that the emotional phases of the change process resemble those of the grieving process identified by Kubler Ross (1970). Some of the reasons for this are as follows:

- preference for stability
- habit conformity
- threat to self-interest (prestige, economic, etc.)
- misunderstanding
- contradictory values
- low change tolerance
- fear of the unknown.

Resistance to change, on the one hand, could be seen as important in order for change not to progress too quickly and it allows for assumptions to the proposed change to be reviewed and analysed more thoroughly. On the other hand, it poses additional difficulties for innovation and creativity to be taken on board by the change agents.

Much bureaucracy within the health service often holds up change for improvement as decisions for change may be required to go through a variety of structures for approval. Bennis (1969) called for more flexible organisations (such as 'adhocracies') to counteract the faults of bureaucracies that can not deal with the rate of rapid change within the increasingly complex organisations. Similarly, Burns and Stalker (1966, 1996) also related that a change in favour of more 'organic' organisational life is needed. This involves more creative and innovative ways of dealing quickly and effectively with problems, which are more easily accepted within the organisational team.

> Think about any new forms of records that have been introduced into your clinical area. Write down what you think influenced their acceptance and/or rejection, noting which issues you think had more force or strength.

Havelock and Huberman (1978) identified several factors that influence acceptance of an innovation (of thought and action):

1. *A sense of ownership* is vital. This can be achieved by their active participation in both formulation and implementation of innovation.
2. *Informal personal contracts* about the innovation as well as formal roles to help reinforce the ownership of the change.
3. *Involvement of opinion leaders:* characteristically, opinion leaders are intelligent, well motivated, enthusiastic about good ideas, articulate and able to deviate from the group norms without losing credibility.
4. *Information and support:* users should be provided with adequate information and support during all stages of the innovation. They should also be helped to see the possibility for personal and professional growth resulting from change and given support to learn any necessary new skill.

This seems to fit well with other theories on managing people in the change process. Upton and Brooks (1995) more recently concur with these ideas and identify the following techniques to gain commitment to change and thus reduce resistance:

- involvement
- visioning
- communication
- 'treating what hurts'
- addressing the readiness and capability of individuals to change
- encouraging people to develop new relationships.

In seeing new care pathways introduced, in one clinical area, staff felt that they were unacceptable. This was because the staff had not all been involved in the design or consultation of the paperwork. The idea was not sold to them and they felt it was imposed. In practice, they communicated this dissatisfaction readily to the patients. This is sad, as documentation is not a problem that should be transferred to patients. Patient surveys showed that patients often complained about the overload of the work of the nurse with the new imposed paperwork.

It is useful to consider the ability of people to 'move' with new ideas when managing a change project. How can you get the people involved to own the change? It would be easy to leave the resisters out of the planning stage but this would have a negative impact on those people, who would distrust the change even more. It would seem that the best way is to acknowledge that the power of communication is vital and should never be underestimated. Involving as many techniques to 'sell' the change will be required and opinions of everyone involved should be taken on board. Exploring 'what hurts' with various people will help you to hear their concerns and to readjust the plans and negotiate a way forward. It is incumbent upon management to take cognisance of factors that will reduce and/or obviate the potential side effects of any change. Any negative energy could be transformed into positive energy as those involved will find that their problems are essentially the same, and they may hold a shared vision of how things could be improved through the proposed change.

Critical care pathways have been brought into some clinical areas, in line with commissioning requirements.

- Consider this situation in your own clinical area and identify who the key people would be.
- Write down who might be the resisters and who might be keen to take on board the change.
- Write down four ways in which you could involve these people.

It could be that different members of staff have a particular clinical interest and it would be useful if they started to draw up standardised care plans within their interest area. Another way could be to ask some people to present the advantages and disadvantages of care pathways. Additionally, someone could attend a conference and then present a report. One other way may be to conduct a trial with the use of pre-set critical pathways for a group of patients and after a period of time get a group together to brainstorm the issues raised during the trial period.

Within any team there will be a variety of behaviours exhibited when there is impending change and innovation. People within a team or organisation may fall into one of the categories listed below, which is adapted from Rogers and Shoemaker (1971):

Change (progressivism)

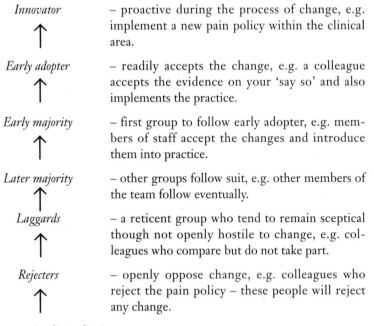

Innovator	– proactive during the process of change, e.g. implement a new pain policy within the clinical area.
Early adopter	– readily accepts the change, e.g. a colleague accepts the evidence on your 'say so' and also implements the practice.
Early majority	– first group to follow early adopter, e.g. members of staff accept the changes and introduce them into practice.
Later majority	– other groups follow suit, e.g. other members of the team follow eventually.
Laggards	– a reticent group who tend to remain sceptical though not openly hostile to change, e.g. colleagues who compare but do not take part.
Rejecters	– openly oppose change, e.g. colleagues who reject the pain policy – these people will reject any change.

Status quo (traditionalism)

Adapted from Rogers and Shoemaker (1971)

This may seem quite simplistic and characterises team members into the good and the bad, let alone the ugly! It is important to see that the various roles are important in taking change forward at the right pace and respect for various diverse views adds to the creativity of change. Otherwise, too rapid and enthusiastic a change, based on one point of view, reflects a 'cloned perspective' which can ultimately be dangerous.

Some questions you might like to ask are:
- Which behavioural pattern do I most often adopt in response to change?
- Is this pattern similar to my friends and family?
- Does my behaviour always fit this pattern or has the pattern changed throughout my life?
- If so, what life events have altered how I view and respond to change?

Refer back to your life map. It is usually dependent on the situation so do not be surprised if you identify differing attributes at different times.

Conclusion

This chapter has offered a brief description of a number of change theories and has attempted to apply them to nursing, midwifery and health visiting. The nature of change was addressed together with the idea that change is inevitable. Lewin's (1951) model was briefly described. While utilising the idea of a 'life map' of changes, personal implications, coping mechanisms and outcomes can be linked to various theories. It was also noted that professional implications of change within work teams may result in zealous behaviour through to resistance and apathy which will ultimately affect the success of the change. Organisational change requires long-term approaches and various models of successful change strategies were highlighted. The skills of successful change agents (such as nurses, midwives and health visitors) were put in the context of planning and managing change. The need to recognise the pain and fear involved in change was seen to be a feature of personal, team and organisational change and should not be underestimated.

Summary of key points

This chapter has examined the following areas:

- **The nature of change:** Was seen to be an inevitable fact of life but caused fear and misunderstanding, as there is a tendency for preferring stability. Imposed change caused most fear.

- **The change process:** Involved 'unfreezing' the old mindset, introducing new ideas and attitudes and 'freezing' the new mindset.

- **Nurses, midwives and health visitors as change agents:** Links in the empowering idea that these professionals have *opportunities* to effect change for the benefits of their patients and clients rather than having change imposed upon them.

- **Change agent skills:** Involved communicating future visions, involving people and encouraging information sharing about the fear within supportive environments. Skills involve being a problem seeker, problem solver, innovator and leader.

- **Planning and managing effective change:** Involved the use of various methods such as force field analysis to anticipate difficulties as well as the need to bring on board appropriate catalysts for change and to recognise that the pace of change may be long term. Approaches such as empirical – rational and normative – re-educative were seen as acceptable and developmental ways for successful long-term change.

References

Armstrong M (1990) *How to Be an Even Better Manager*, Kogan Page

Bennis W G (1969) *Organizational Development: Its Nature, Origins and Prospects*, Addison-Wesley

Burke W W (1982) *Organisational Development: Principles and Practice*, Little, Brown.

Burns T and Stalker G M (1966) *The Management of Innovation*, Tavistock

Burns T and Stalker G M (1996) *The Management of Innovation* (2nd edn), Tavistock

Chinn R (1988) in Bennis W, Benne K D and Chinn R (eds) The planning of change, in Parsley K and Corrigan P (1999) *Quality Improvement in Healthcare: Putting Evidence into Practice* (2nd edn) Stanley Thornes

Clarke J E and Copcutt L (1997) *Management for Nurses and Health Care Professionals*, Churchill Livingstone

Gray H L (1985) *Change and Management in Schools*, Deanhouse

Handy C B (1985) *Understanding Organizations* (3rd edn) Penguin Business

Havelock R G and Huberman A M (1978) *Solving Educational Problems: The Theory and Reality of Innovation in Developing Countries*, Praeger, Holt, Reinhart & Winston

Huczynski A and Buchanan D (1991) *Organisation Behaviour* (2nd edn), Prentice Hall

Iles V (1997) *Really Managing Health Care*, Open University

Kubler Ross E (1970) *On Death and Dying*, Tavistock Publications

Lewin K (1951) *Field Theory in Social Sciences*, Harper & Row

Peters T and Waterman R (1995) *In Search of Excellence* HarperCollins

Rogers E and Shoemaker F (1971) *Communication of Innovations: A Cross-cultural Report*, The Free Press

Tappen R M (1995) *Nursing Leadership and Management* (3rd edn) F A Davis

Teasdale K (1992) *Managing the Changes in Health Care*, Wolfe

Upton T and Brooks B (NAHAT) (1995) *Managing Change in the NHS*, Kogan Page

UKCC (1999) *Making a Difference: The Contribution of Nursing, Midwifery and Health Visiting*, UKCC

van der Peet R (1995) *The Nightingale Model of Nursing*, Campion Press

Further reading

Bass L J and Wood K M (1987) Nurses can change things, *Nursing*, **17**(10),47–8

Bowman M (1995) *The Professional Nurse Coping with Change: Now and the Future*, Chapman & Hall

Broome A (1990) *Managing Change*, Macmillan

Department of Health (1999) *Making a Difference: The Contribution of Nursing, Midwifery and Health Visiting*, The Stationery Office

Field P A (1989) Implementing change in nursing education, *Nurse Education Today*, **9**(5), 290–9

Kadner K (1984) Change: introducing computer assisted instruction (CAI) to a college of nursing faculty, *Journal of Nursing Education*, **23**(8), 349–50

Lancaster J (1999) *Nursing Issues in Leading and Managing Change*, Mosby

King M L (1963) in Microsoft Encarta 97 (World English Edition)

Marquis B L and Huston C J (1996) *Leadership Roles and Management Functions in Nursing: Theory & Application* (2nd edn) Lippincott

McKenna E (1994) *Business Psychology & Organisational Behaviour: A Students' Handbook*, Lawrence Erlbaum Associates.

Mullins L J (1989) *Management and Organisational Behaviour* (2nd edn) Pitman

Northcott N (1989) Workshops to manage change. *Nursing (London): The Journal of Clinical Practice, Education & Management*, 3(47), 26–7

Paton R and McCalman (2000) *Change Management: A Guide to Effective Implementation*, (2nd edn) Sage

Perlman D and Takacs G J (1990), The ten stages of change, *Nursing Management*, 21(4), 33–8

Sheehan J (1990) Investigating change in a nursing context, *Journal of Advanced Nursing*, 15(7), 819–24

Stephenson P M (1987) The process of change in intensive care nursing, *Intensive Care Nursing* 2(4), 148-56

Sullivan E J and Decker P J (1997) *Effective Leadership and Management in Nursing*, (4th edn) Addison Wesley

Teasdale K (1992) *Managing the Changes in Health Care*, Wolfe

Upton T and Brooks B (NAHAT) (1995) *Managing change in the NHS*, Kogan Page

Wright S (1993) The Standard guide to ... achieving change quietly, *Nursing Standard*, 7(26), 52-4

Wright S G (ed.) (1998) *Changing Nursing Practice* (2nd edn) Arnold

Part

III

The business of health care

9

The business of health

By the end of this chapter you will have had the opportunity to:

- identify the historical picture of the management of health services in Britain
- recognise the impact of recent health policies
- discuss the implications of the new and modern health service for nurses, midwives and health visitors.

Introduction

As we continue to examine the wider perspectives of managing in health care it is important that we recognise the impact of government policies on the management and delivery of that care. The purpose of this chapter is to highlight the impact of social, economic and political factors on the business of health service provision and allow you to relate this to professional practice.

The context of managing health services

Health is valued in most societies, whether rich or poor. However, the way that different governments across the world allocate resources to their health services reflects diverse problems and settings for health care. There are certain common factors that influence the evolution of health care systems in all countries (Muir Gray 1997). There are typical demographical, technological and sociological elements affecting all countries. A minister for health in a Third World country is responsible for providing appropriate services to deal not only with the typical Third World problems such as high infant mortality rates and infection control but also with the consequences of Western influences such as cigarette smoking, drug abuse and dangerous driving, which are considered part of twentieth-century living. Technological advances across the world have been made and are being introduced to Third World countries but may only be available to a small population in that country. There are therefore *common* health service problems and *common* solutions are being sought.

The common features are as follows:

- a need for cost control
- the ability to develop systems to prevent health costs falling on the individual
- authority being given to 'purchaser function' to cover a certain geographical area or members of a certain health plan or fund
- defining and delineating the purchasing function from central government to an agency/agencies
- an increasing appreciation of the need to manage the evolution of clinical practice along with professionals
- increasing public interest in evidence for effectiveness and efficiency. (Muir Gray 1997)

Taking Muir Gray's ideas forward, write some notes about how you feel about each of the above points and whether you think they are important to clinical care:

- across the world
- in this country.

Clearly, you might say there is a case for cost control wherever you are. It is not good policy to spend unnecessarily; indeed, think of your own expenses and what happens if you are not aware of the price of things or if you 'impulse buy' – you can get into all kinds of financial trouble. So budget management is something that affects people both across the world and in this country. You might have thought of the history of the health service in Britain and one of its main features is that care is free at the point of delivery. If this is to remain the case then there must be some system in place to prevent costs falling on the individual. In Britain this is through the taxation/National Insurance system. In countries where the delivery of health care is not free, then there are usually insurance plans in place for the individual to buy into in order to cover any costs. For example, in the United States the common belief is that introducing competition will induce the cheapest services, so maintaining cost effectiveness. You will have to consider which system you prefer! One can continue doing this for each of the points that Muir Gray raised but overall it can be seen that for each of these points there are advantages and disadvantages.

The World Health Organization (WHO) has been instrumental in putting health on the agenda for all countries and attempts to support the development of health care systems to raise the health potential of all peoples worldwide. The WHO's *Health For All* strategy (World Health Organization 1985) in the 1980s is based on the premise of health need assessment and action.

Health care in Britain

The NHS was started in 1948, after the Second World War, by the Minister of Health, Aneurin Bevin, and it demonstrated a particularly idealistic view of reforming the welfare state and combating the evils of disease and poverty. The effects of the Industrial Revolution had long caused concern which had been raised by anti-poverty activists such as Edwin Chadwick (1800–90), Charles Booth (1840–1916) and Seebohm Rowntree (1871–1954) in the public domain. The economic depression of the 1930s had highlighted particular problems in health, housing and social welfare. However, the NHS ideal, set out by the Beveridge Report of 1942 and agreed by the then Coalition Government, was not accepted immediately and there was well-documented resistance from the British Medical Association (BMA) which required careful handling. The proposed comprehensive health service was based on a set of underlying principles including the notion of a service 'free at the point of delivery'. Seedhouse (1994) identifies that the ideals of compassion, equity and collective responsibility were enshrined in the four basic principles:

1. Meeting needs.
2. Equity.
3. Access to the best service.
4. Containment of health costs.

It is these four principles that are still at the root of tensions surrounding debates on health care provision. Depending on the political ideology of the times and the socio-economic circumstances, one or more of the principles may dominate and cause concern over the others (Wilkinson 1995). Health policy is where ideology is turned into broad plans for the distribution of a variety of finite resources to meet the needs of the population. Policy takes various forms – reports, Green Papers, White Papers and Acts. In the 1980s it appeared that the budget for health services focused on allocating resources based on 'need' and that measuring costs and outcomes was particularly important. This dominant ideology of both Margaret Thatcher in the UK and Ronald Reagan in the USA meant that there was a focus on libertarian ideals with an emphasis on individual responsibility and the need to decentralise the health service through market reforms (Maynard 1993, p. 58).

The NHS and Community Care Act 1990

The NHS and Community Care Act (1990) was brought about because of the perceived need for radical changes in health care provision in Great Britain. Complex social, economic and political forces highlighted that the NHS could not survive in the same way that it had over the past fifty years.

> Jot down what you think were some of the social, economic and political pressures on the health service that the Conservative Government had to address at that time.

The pressures were the demographic changes of an increasingly elderly population and a reduction in the economically active sector, the pressure of technological advances in biomedics and increasing consumer and thus cost expectations in the health service.

Changes in the health service

The key innovation by the reforms of the Act was the separation of purchasing from the provision of health care services. This led to the setting up of the internal market within the administrative structures, and health authorities, social service departments and GP fundholders had responsibilities to assess health needs and to negotiate with providers for efficient and effective services to meet those needs. This new public management ideology was meant to drive down costs and maximise clinical effectiveness. The health service monopolies were thus challenged in order to control the biomedical dominance and also open up more consumer choice through primary care structures, involving the private and voluntary sectors. The internal market altered the power bases dramatically within health care, through changed structures and processes of the service; even within nursing and midwifery there was self-interest and interprofessional conflict rather than patient focus. So how did the internal market affect patient care? It certainly opened the public's eyes to rationing and inefficiency. Patients undergoing surgery and receiving maternity or mental health care experienced shorter in-patient stays, long-term medical care was moved to a 'means-tested' social care basis and much money went into letterheads, carpets and signposts rather than staffing, pillows or mouthwash tablets!

However, in the community, there was an increase in district nursing and practice nursing posts and an overwhelming growth in administrative structures to support the new focus. More patients were seen by community nurses and midwives but most of the burden of care was placed within the community through family, kinship and voluntary structures. Robinson and Le Grand (1994) found that fundholding was a key aspect of the Act which affected the competitive efficiency of hospitals in the way the reformers had hoped. This statement relates to the fact that the ethos of fundholding was the biggest impetus for changes within the acute or hospital care delivery system. So when it was known that care was to be 'purchased', suddenly questions were asked as to whether a particular form of treatment was actually required or whether there was an alternative. Thus it was the community provision via GPs and others that affected the acute sector rather than the other way around. The uptake of fundholding by some GPs was variable in particular areas. Some felt that the bureaucracy attached to fundholding would compromise their clinical practice.

The Labour Government and the Health Act 1999

The latest reforms under New Labour recently have not in themselves dramatically reversed the NHS and Community Care Act but they demonstrate a focus on quality over cost with the branding of modernisation. The 1997 White Paper *The New NHS, Modern, Dependable* (Department of Health 1997) therefore refocused the health service in a different way from the 1990 Act. The questions to ask now are:

- How does current health policy affect health?
- How does curreny health policy affect health care provision?
- How does current health policy affect nursing?

Jot down some ideas from your own knowledge about the answers to these questions.

Let us now discuss the issues you might have thought of under the three headings:

- health policy and health,
- health policy and health care provision (linking this to the National Performance Framework)
- health policy linked to nursing, midwifery and health visiting.

Health policy and health

It has to be recognised that health services alone do not secure health. Health in itself is considered an elusive concept, incorporating the facets of physical, mental, social and spiritual harmony. The Western world's focus on the physical aspects of health has often been equated with the need for services to meet the dominant physical disorders. Hennessy and Spurgeon (2000, p. 3) highlight that the social context of individual health may have more influence over health than purely the health services. Housing, education and meaningful employment within the context of peace are as vital to health as the statutory health service provision. Therefore health policy, as a means of distributing finite resources to meet infinite need, must be seen in the context of all social policy.

Health policy and health care provision

All new health policy makes changes to the way that health needs and services are matched. The main changes they make are:

- changes to the perception of health needs
- changes to health care structures and systems
- changes to health care processes
- changes to roles and responsibilities
- changes to power bases
- challenges to the *status quo*.

> Think about a recent policy/Act and write down how it may have affected any of the points above.

You may have thought about nurse prescribing (The Medicinal Products: Prescription by Nurses etc. Act, 1992). The patients can now be seen by a district nurse and have their prescription delivered at the same time rather than requiring them to wait for a doctor to sign the prescription. Systems, structures and processes are thus much simpler, district nurse roles and responsibilities are greater through their increased powerbase and the status quo within the Primary Health Care Team (PHCT) is challenged.

For mental health nurses the Mental Health Act (1983) is being revised and reformed. Within the 1983 Act, section 5(4) was important: This is, also known as the 'nurses' holding power' section, whereby patients who are a potential danger to themselves or others, and who have been receiving treatment for a mental disorder, may be held for up to six hours or until the medical officer arrives. The consultation exercise found that '91% of people and organisations who responded to the issue wanted the ward manager (nurses') holding power of six hours to be retained' (Department of Health 2000c). This evidence supports the findings of Ward (1991) who stated that in her survey 85–90 per cent of mental health trained nurses found it useful and those who did not find it useful gave the following reasons:

- too much responsibility for an RMN
- too much trouble for only six hours.

The structures and processes are still in place but some are in the process of being updated. Roles and responsibilities are being addressed while retaining the powerbase for the registered practitioner in the areas of mental health and learning difficulty.

For midwives you may have considered the changing childbirth policy (Department of Health 1993) whereby the notion of the named midwife was to be implemented, thus enabling the client to experience continuity of care throughout her pregnancy, delivery and during the post-natal period. In theory this was an excellent idea although it did seem to resemble the past when community midwives were 'on call' for their patients within a specific area. However, in practice it would require additional funding and additional midwives to meet the clients' expectations. Unfortunately, due to the lack of resources, it could be said that the Act did not affect care in the way it was envisaged and so disappeared into oblivion. Had it been fully implemented it would have further empowered not only the midwives but the clients also.

The New Labour Government wanted to depict its modernisation as the 'Third Way' regarding health care provision in order to make the organisation more effective and efficient. To this end the paper *The New NHS, Modern, Dependable* (Department of Health 1997) was a major force in the development of health care delivery and developed into the Health Act 1999. The principles of the Act were as follows:

- to renew the NHS as a genuinely national service
- to make the delivery of health care against new national standards a matter of local responsibility
- to get the NHS to work in partnership
- to improve efficiency
- to move the focus onto quality of care so that excellence is guaranteed
- to rebuild public confidence.

Its aims were to shape the NHS into the next millennium through, the following:

- commissioning rather than purchasing
- competition replaced with cooperation
- development of primary care groups from total fundholding
- setting up health improvement programmes
- clinical governance and quality standards
- health action zones to be identified
- the introduction of technology in the form of NHS Direct and NHS Net.

Jot down your own ideas about how much you know about these changes and whether you feel the Act has achieved any of its aims.

The National Service Framework

Within these ideas, the focus was on efficiency and performance with changing roles for health authorities and Trusts and primary care groups. Areas of performance were set into National Service Frameworks which included set standards and focused on measuring health outcomes against the standards across the country and between various Trusts.

Do you know of any National Service Framework areas? Some of the areas relate to coronary heart disease and vascular diseases, accidents, surgery and mental health. The setting up of these 'league tables' is a 'hot potato' for debate today. It could be said that there are three main reasons for using performance league tables in the health service:

1. To ensure that NHS goals are achieved.
2. To be accountable to a growing range of stakeholders.
3. To survive through competition.

It could be said that this third reason is not particularly apparent within the Labour Government's agenda but it does not seem to be rational for league tables to be thus published. In terms of efficiency and effectiveness in performance, the following notions may help you to expand your ideas about health service quality. Quality initiatives such as clinical governance were put in place, and structures such as the National Institute of Clinical Excellence (NICE) and the Commission for Health Improvement (CHI) were created in order to review effective treatments within the country.

Jot down how you think these changes affected:
- the perception of health needs
- health care structures and systems
- health care processes
- roles and responsibilities
- powerbases
- the *status quo*.

People are becoming far more health aware and so health needs are changing. Together with this, increased longevity of the population is making greater demands on health care provision, requiring increased resources. In terms of structures and systems there is greater input into community care with patients being discharged earlier from acute areas. There are a greater number of elderly people requiring ongoing care in the community; mental health patients are also moving into community care settings as we see the demise of the large mental health and learning difficulty institutions. Roles and responsibilities are changing with the inception of nurse prescribing, single drugs administration and nurses being able to undertake minor surgical procedures (with appropriate training), e.g. suturing. Most health policy shapes what is seen to be important in terms of ill health. The need to find out what is effective, what is measurable and what is preventable appear admirable motives. Physical problems such as cancer, heart disease, strokes and accidents as well as overall surgical cures are, to a large extent, valued as areas to measure. Depression and suicide are also seen as relatively important issues that need to be measured and prevented. However, there are many health problems that are considered less important and they tend to be the needs that are difficult to quantify, prevent and cure, for example multiple sclerosis, drug addiction, Alzheimer's disease and even the problem of incontinence. In these areas biomedicine is not always successful, and care is the basic need. We now seem to have a health service for health *cure* rather than health *care*.

The Health Act again has changed the very substance of the NHS system. Greater emphasis is being placed on setting up new management structures such as primary care groups and Trusts. Interestingly, the structure of primary care is set to become more complex, and access to a variety of primary care providers is being widened. This is useful in widening access to health services such as:

- various models of general practice such as personal medical services (PMS)
- NHS Direct
- one-stop health shops.

The benefits for patients are stated to be that they will be able to get easier and faster advice and information. Systems for referral will also be changed with the use of the NHS Net to link primary and acute care more tightly. Exciting developments are being tested to improve the present systems of health care. Palfrey (2000, p. 131) notes that hospital appointments, if appropriate, will be booked while the patient waits in consultation and hospital test results will be despatched electronically to the doctor's screen. Telemedicine will play an increasingly significant role in the diagnosis and treatment of patients. This is already in place within the emergency services where information can be sent directly to the Accident & Emergency Department prior to the arrival of the patient so that advice can be given during the transportation of the patient. In diagnostics, information can be sent directly from the GP surgery to the acute unit in order to ensure that the patient can access correct treatment sooner. Together with this, the focus on waiting lists and performance will also mean that patients should be seen and treated more quickly. There are pledges that patients with cancer problems will be seen within two weeks by a specialist.

Roles of professionals are being affected by this shaping of the health service. Primary care generalist roles are required and more GPs/nurses with management experience are required. Specialist doctors and nurses with experience, especially in 'high dependency' total care management are needed. More flexible roles are required to deliver quality care to the increasing number of dependent groups. *A Workforce for All Talents* (Department of Health 2000a) highlights the importance of the various roles and indeed nursing, midwifery and health visiting figure very importantly in *The NHS Plan* (Department of Health 2000b) which sets out to realise the objectives of the Health Act 2000.

The powerbases across the NHS have definitely been challenged, and community and primary care are no longer seen as 'Cinderella' services. This has obviously affected the *status quo* of personnel within the health service and recognition and rewards need to follow suit.

Primary care groups and Trusts

The strategic change to a primary care-led NHS is not yet clearly defined, particularly as primary care groups (PCGs) develop towards Trust status. PCG and Trusts will be making some important decisions about health service provision for their local populations. They will be able to commission (shape and 'buy') various contracts of health service. These PCGs and Trusts are relatively inexperienced and, in many cases, there will be role conflict between managing services and providing clinical care. The tensions between a bottom-up approach to developing services to meet needs and the priorities previously set by health authorities may lead to greater fragmentation of policy. Hunter (1996) feels that primary care developments could emerge 'on the hoof', and although this is not necessarily problematic there is a need for clear understanding and communication about the evolving health policy. Hunter, however, highlights the real problem that primary care can never really succeed until the interface between health and social care has been addressed. This is where health policy affects public health agendas.

Health improvement: the regeneration of public health

Public health within the health service is an important branch of the NHS but has not always been seen as integral to the total service. Public health has developed over time:

- public health movement 1840s–1920s
- health education era 1920s–1970s

- health promotion 1940s–1990s
- new public health 1980s–2000: Labour's 'Third Way' approach.

Health action zones (HAZs) and the health improvement programmes (HIMPs) are now set within the scene of the new public health movement and the Health Act 1999.

> For all those charged with planning and providing health and social care services for patients will work to a jointly agreed Health Improvement Programme. This will govern the actions of all parts of the local NHS to ensure consistency and coordination. (Department of Health 1997)

The White Paper (Department of Health 1999a) entitled *Our Healthier Nation – Saving Lives* illustrated that poverty, unemployment, bad housing and social isolation were major determinants of health and illness and focused on various 'action settings':

- healthy schools
- workplaces
- neighbourhoods.

HAZs are now identified for extra funding to improve the health of those populations. There are four priority areas that are set within the HIPs:

1. Coronary heart disease /stroke.
2. Cancers.
3. Accidents.
4. Mental health.

HIMPs are seen as part of the local needs assessment and planning process that will be developed by the NHS, local authorities and others, including the public, to improve health and health care. These programmes should address the following:

- the health needs of the local population
- the main health care requirements of local people and how local services will be developed
- the range location and investment required in local health services.

They will also place increased emphasis on the effectiveness of health-promoting interventions and will need to be integrated into the plans of each PCG/T. *The Acheson Report* (Department of Health 1999b) reinforced the inequality issues within our populations and showed how the gap between rich and poor was still widening. Transport, good education, housing and employment are seen to be the elements that exclude people socially from accessing health services. It is hoped that HIMPs and HAZs will address the social exclusion problems within our communities, but long- rather than short-term planning and investment will be required for sustainable change amidst a biomedical emphasis in health care.

Nursing, midwifery and health visiting

The focus on primary care will continue and there is a need for nursing and midwifery to think and respond in new ways. There will be opportunities for them:

- to search for new scientific knowledge to underpin and account for practice
- to be able to develop more flexible and effective skills
- to be involved in commissioning
- to participate in drawing up HIMPs, focusing on outcomes and addressing inequalities
- greater inter-agency working across health authority and local authority boundaries – geographical focus
- to be expected to provide integrated care across primary and secondary care
- to expand the range of nursing and midwifery in primary care
- to lead within the NHS Direct
- to be increasingly responsible for quality and efficiency of their service
- to shift from counting the numbers to measuring quality
- to participate in profiling, public health and making recommendations.

However, these are not easy challenges and the skills are not necessarily there. If there is no strength in the nursing and midwifery powerbase, they will be sidelined and a new bureaucracy will take their roles. There are plenty of others who are not health care professionals – general managers, politicians and private IT companies, to name a few – who feel that they know about health needs and are already getting into commissioning and nurses are being left out. Nurses and midwives have long been apolitical but these are times when they need to push themselves into the public arena and grasp the new opportunities to rebalance the inequalities of health care provision.

Conclusion

This chapter has examined a variety of influences that affect the provision and delivery of health care in Britain. Government policy together with technological, demographic and sociological factors all impact on the delivery of health care. In the context of managing health services we noted Muir Gray's writings on the evolution of health care systems throughout the world and how they affect such things as mortality rates. Changes within the British system were then addressed, examining the effects on health policy, care provision, NICE, PCGs and Trusts together with the effort to regenerate public health through HAZs and HIMPs and the focus on primary care. These points all serve to demonstrate the complexity of health care delivery.

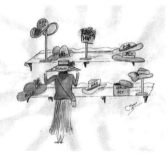

Summary of key points

This chapter has examined the following areas:

- **The context of managing health services:** Health is valued in most societies but there are differing ways of meeting these needs across the world. The common feature of meeting these needs is that of cost and effectiveness.

- **Health care in Britain:** The NHS came into existence in 1948 in order to combat the evils of disease and poverty and the focus of today's NHS is still that care should be free at the point of delivery.

- **The NHS and Community Care Act:** This Act was brought about because of the perceived need for radical changes in health care provision.

- **Changes in the health service:** The key reforms of the Health Act 1999 led to the changes outlined within this section. Increasing technology played a major role in the changes together with demographic changes which meant that there was a greater demand on resources.

- **Health policy and health care provision:** The changes related to a variety of Acts and policies were discussed, linking them to adult and mental health nursing together with midwifery practice.

- **The National Performance Framework:** Here we examined quality issues, linking them to NICE and CHI together with how these bodies affected health needs, structures, processes, roles, responsibilities and the powerbase.

- **Primary care groups and Trusts:** Here we demonstrated a move towards a 'new' management approach whereby groups of people are charged with 'commissioning' contracts of health service provision.

- **Nursing, Midwifery and Health Visiting:** The focus on primary care continues and highlights the need for nursing, midwifery and health visisting to respond in new ways in order to meet the challenges of the 21st century.

References

Department of Health (1993) *Vision for the Future*, HMSO

Department of Health (1997) *The New NHS, Modern, Dependable*, The Stationery Office

Department of Health (1999a) *Our Healthier Nation – Saving Lives*, The Stationery Office

Department of Health (1999b) *The Acheson Report*, The Stationery Office

Department of Health (2000a) *A Health Service of All Talents*, The Stationery Office

Department of Health (2000b) *The NHS Plan*, The Stationery Office

Department of Health (2000c) *Reform of the Mental Health Act 1983*, The Stationery Office

Hennessy D and Spurgeon P (2000) *Health Policy and Nursing*, Palgrave

Hunter D (1996) *Health Policy Overview: National Association for Health Authorities and Trusts NHS handbook*

Maynard A (1993) Creating competition in the NHS: is it possible? Will it work?, in Tilley I (ed.) *Managing the Internal Market*, Paul Chapman Publishing

Muir Gray J A (1997) *Evidence-based Healthcare*, Churchill Livingstone

Palfrey C (2000) *Key Concepts in Healthcare Policy and Planning*

Robinson R and Le Grand J (1994) *Evaluating the NHS Reforms*, King's Fund Institute

Seedhouse D (1994) *Fortress NHS: A Philosophical Review of the NHS*, Wiley

Ward J (1991) How useful is Section 5(4)?, *Nursing Times*, **87** (27)

Wilkinson M J (1995) Love is not a marketable commodity: new public management in the British National Health Service, *Journal of Advanced Nursing*, **21** (5), 980 – 7

World Health Organization (1985) *Health for All by the Year 2000*, WHO

Further reading

Allott M and Robb M (1998) *Understanding Health and Social Care*, Sage/Open University

Department of Health (1998) *A First Class Service: Quality in the New NHS*, The Stationery Office

Department of Health (1999) *Making a Difference: Strengthening the Nursing, Midwifery and Health Visiting Contribution to Health and Health Care*, The Stationery Office

Ham C (1998) The organization of the NHS, in Merry P (ed.) *1998/1999 NHS Handbook* (13th edn) JMH Publishing

Opit L (1993) Commissioning: an appraisal of a new role in Tilley I (ed.) *Managing the Internal Market*, Paul Chapman Publishing

10

Quality in health care

By the end of this chapter you will have had the opportunity to:

● recognise the concepts and models of quality assurance in the context of contemporary health care.
● discuss the developments of quality in Britain
● evaluate the present quality framework for health care
● draw out the implications for nursing and midwifery.

Introduction

In order to guarantee an excellent service one has to be cognisant of all aspects of quality. This chapter will examine the overall concept of quality that which was introduced into the British system from abroad, total quality management, customer care and government papers, e.g. *A First Class Service: Quality in the New NHS Health Services* (Department of Health 1998). Together with these, this chapter will also examine the concepts of clinical governance, clinical audit, clinical effectiveness, clinical risk management and quality assurance. Finally these factors will be related to their impact on staff development and how this enhances the overall quality of care delivery to the patients/clients in the system.

Concept of quality

Quality is a relative concept and although we all have some idea of what is good and what is bad, it is not so simple to identify what is acceptable. The British Standards Institute defines quality, as 'the totality of features and characteristics of a product or service that bears on its ability to satisfy stated or applied needs'. This is particularly true for a health care service, just as it is for a car industry or for the holiday business. Being effective and efficient in any business is the basis for success. Drucker (1967) defined efficiency simply as 'doing things right' and effectiveness as 'doing the right things right'. The questions to ask are 'what is right?' and 'how do we know we are doing them right?' However, effectiveness and efficiency may not tell the full story of quality tensions in health care. Øvretveit (1992) defines quality in health services as 'fully meeting requirements of lowest cost or more specifically fully meeting the needs of those who need the service most at the lowest cost to the organisation within the limits and directives set by higher authorities and purchasers'. The question of defining quality is difficult and it is probably more important to focus on the elements of quality.

The World Health Organization (1983) identified the four main principles of quality assurance in heath care:

1. Professional performance (technical quality).
2. Resource use (efficiency).
3. Risk management.
4. Patient satisfaction with the service provided.

Developments on the world stage of quality health care have been captured by the work of the World Health Organization. In 1985 the WHO working party on quality reported four central features behind the interest in this phenomenon:

1. *Political*: There are political pressures to make services more like markets and to construct patients as customers. Ideas from business and commerce may be used to hide a fall in standards.
2. *Economic*: Resources cannot keep pace with rising demands and expectations.
3. *Social*: People are less likely to accept poor quality in health care and may be more likely to sue.
4. *Professional*: Health professions generally want to do their best for their patients and clients.

Different governments across the world allocate different amounts of their Gross National Product to health provision. Table 10.1 illustrates, over time and place, the differing values that are placed on health care by governments.

Table 10.1 Expenditure on health care as a percentage of GNP 1960–1998

Country	1960	1970	1980	1987	1992	1997–8
Australia	4.6	5.0	6.5	7.1	8.2	N/A
Italy	3.3	4.8	6.8	6.9	8.1	N/A
Netherlands	3.9	6.0	8.2	8.5	8.9	N/A
Sweden	4.7	7.2	9.5	9.0	7.9	N/A
UK	3.9	4.5	5.8	6.1	7.5	5.6
USA	5.2	7.4	9.2	11.2	13.0	N/A

Quality brought into the health service from abroad

It is only since the 1970s and early 1980s that the concept of quality rather than quantity became more important in industry. Previously, the only reference was perhaps in the context of the old rag trade saying, 'never mind the quality, feel the width'. Quality had begun to be associated with the manufacturing industry where products were *inspected* for their worth. However, this was rarely associated with the service industries and particularly not in health care. Health care was felt to be in the business for altruistic motives rather than profit which was not open for quality scrutiny. One of the views of quality development in all organisational life can be seen from Table 10.2.

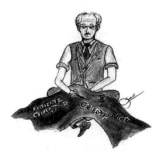

Table 10.2 Development of quality frameworks

	Traditional pre-1960	**Technocratic 1960s and 1970s**	**TQM 1980s and 1990s**
Definition	*La crème de la crème*	Fitness for use and meeting requirements	Satisfying and delighting the customer
Who defines quality?	Everybody knows what it is	Experts	Customers
Nature of quality	Attributes of product or service	Attributes of product or service	Process and outcomes
What produces good quality?	Good people and materials	Good people and materials	The right processes
Relationship to cost	Top quality is the most expensive	Quality can be found at all prices but improving quality implies raising costs	Quality is free

Context of quality movement in the health service

It was in 1984 that the British government launched the National Quality Campaign for both private and public industries and the NHS was strongly encouraged to ensure a quality control system. There was initial resistance and scepticism from professionals who felt that they already gave a quality service. From these initial developments, the NHS worked through concepts such as quality assurance (which assured a quality) to the total quality management (TQM) concept (which focuses on a quality organisation meeting and satisfying the needs of customers) and the now more fashionable concept of continuous process improvement. The latter idea focuses on an active journey of not only meeting customer needs but on delighting the customer. The Patient's Charter (Department of Health 1991) set down precise national standards for health care, which were incorporated into a quality strategy in health care. More recently the Health Act 1999 focused on the quality of health care through the instigation of a National Performance Framework, clinical governance and quality structures such as the National Institute for Clinical Excellence (NICE) and the Commission for Health Improvement (CHI). The policy document *A First Class Service* (Department of Health 1998) made more specific plans for progress in improving the health service, especially in terms of effectiveness, efficiency and excellence. The drive for quality is seen through partnership and performance. NICE will be the agency for establishing which overall treatments and interventions work best and making sure that clinicians know about them. CHI will be responsible for monitoring clinical governance and will be able to investigate organisations that fall short of providing adequate care (Garbett 1998). The quality of nursing and midwifery care needs to be seen in the context of all health care provision. We cannot expect to improve nursing and midwifery care if the NHS is not committed to quality improvement as a whole.

Total quality management

Total quality management, introduced very successfully by Deming (1986) to Japan initially in the 1950s, is a business philosophy based on customer satisfaction and requires continuous improvement and is determined by the system (see Table 10.3). TQM is also a business strategy aimed at the whole organisation so that resources are better managed and people cooperate so that the organisation is more flexible and responsive to what are known as internal and external customers. The term 'customers' is considered problematic in health care for many reasons, not least the marketing of health care brought about by the 1990 NHS and Community Care Act. However, the use of the term 'customer' within the concept of quality has a different focus. In thinking about TQM and continuous improvement, all customers have an important role in quality improvement.

Table 10.3 Quality management

Deming identified fourteen points for managing quality in any organisation:

1. Create constancy of purpose for improvement of service.
2. Adopt a new philosophy.
3. Cease dependence upon inspection to achieve quality.
4. End the practice of awarding business on price alone. Instead minimise total cost.

5. Improve constantly and forever every process for planning and service.
6. Institute training on the job
7. Adopt and institute leadership.
8. Drive out fear.
9. Break down barriers between staff areas.
10. Eliminate slogans and targets for the workforce.
11. Eliminate numerical quotas for staff and numerical goals for management.
12. Remove barriers that rob people of pride of workmanship.
13. Institute a vigorous programme of education and self-improvement for everyone.
14. Put everyone to work to accomplish the transformation.

Adapted from Deming (1986)

Customers could be seen as individuals or groups of people to whom you provide one or more product or service. The breadth of this definition means that customers can be our patients and clients, known as *external customers* as they are outside the organisation. Customers can also be anyone or any group with whom we link up in providing a health care service. So as health care professionals we may need to consider path. labs, catering staff, porters and record departments as part of our customer base, as we are theirs. We may need to provide information services to them so that they can provide their services to us. These are known as *internal customers* within an organisation. All internal departments are affected by the quality of each other and that no department/discipline works in isolation. If the salaries department did not come up with their services on time, then all departments would be up in arms! It is also true to say that the other external links are also our customers such as the health or local authority, community health council and voluntary and private sectors as well as the new primary care groups in the community.

A first-class health service

Various ideas of quality health care have been proposed. The Department of Health (1998) publication. *A First Class Service: Quality in the New NHS* reflects the need for clear lines of responsibility and quality management activities incorporating monitoring and continuous improvement. Clinical effectiveness, evidence-based practice, clinical supervision and continuing professional development activities highlight the specific need for first-class health practitioners. Maxwell (1984) introduced a framework of quality into health care which is still recognised as valuable today.

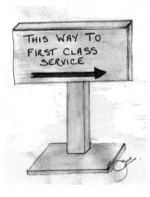

This highlighted the various aspects of quality in health care but very much from a focus of patients as customers:

- *acceptability*
  - services are provided such as to satisfy the reasonable expectations of patients, purchasers, providers and the community
- *equity*
  - a fair share for all the population
  - the service or procedure is what the individual or population actually needs
- *efficiency*
  - resources are not wasted on one service or patient to the detriment of another
- *effectiveness*
  - achieving the intended benefit for the individual and the population
- *accessibility*
  - services are not compromised by undue limits of time or distance.

Jot down your thoughts and feelings about these aspects in relation to your practical experience.

You may feel that these are all important but from time to time there can be difficulties in reaching a good standard of care that meets all these criteria. So what about standards? What do they mean for health practitioners? The setting of local standards of all kinds of care is seen as vital to assuring quality. We hear the phrases 'the standard of care needs to be improved' or 'there is a good standard of care here' so often. The RCN (1988) defined a standard as a 'professionally agreed level of performance appropriate to the population.' Standards should:

- describe the desired quality of performance
- have been agreed
- be clearly written
- contain one major thought
- be measurable
- be concise
- be specific
- be achievable
- be clinically sound.

There are eight prerequisites for a successful standard:

1. A philosophy.
2. The relevant skills and knowledge.
3. The authority to act.

4. Accountability.
5. The control of resources.
6. Organisational structure and management style.
7. The professional relationships.
8. The management of change.

Standard statements should be related, descriptive, free from bias, suitable for quantification, valid and reliable so that they are unambiguous. There have been several quality assurance (QA) models for standard setting proposed and used in nursing. Donabedian's (1966) approach to quality evaluation has been regularly used within the NHS and serves as a reminder of the different domains that affect health care. The Dynamic Standard Setting System (DySSSy) for nursing was based on this approach within the UK:

- *Structure* refers to factors within the organisation that enable work to be carried out such as environmental facilities, equipment, staffing, educational facilities and management
- *Process* refers to performance – the care given to an individual, group or community.
- *Outcome* is the end result of care and performance, the effect of care on an individual, group or community.

Kitson (1988) proposed a cycle of quality assurance that involved three stages:

1. *Describing phase*
   - select topic for quality improvement
   - identify care group
   - identify criteria (structure; process; outcome)
   - agree standard
2. *Measuring Phase*
   - refine criteria
   - select or construct measuring tool
   - collect data
   - evaluate results
3. *Taking Action Phase*
   - consider course of action following results
   - plan action
   - take action
   - re-evaluate results.

This fits in with the 'plan, do and check' cycle which is linked to TQM theories. However, Keighley (1989), argued against the Donabedian approach and identified two elements of a quality standard: the technical performance and the expressive performance. *Technical performance* is something that the customer expects the NHS to deliver consistently. Good technical performance is achieved through knowledge that is required in training, in the use of supplies and the use of facilities and, most of all, is dependent on the number of staff available to deliver the service. In contrast, *expressive performance* is concerned with attitudes of staff towards their relationships and interactions with customers and with each other, and with the manner in which the staff deliver the service.

Expressive performance is therefore more difficult to measure than technical performance. Keighley (1989) goes on to say:

> a customer may experience high quality technical performance and delivery of care, but may be subjected to a poor expressive performance. The overwhelming perception of the customer will be that they have been given a low quality service.

It is also true that this in practice may cloud a patient's/client's view of a health service forever even when different personnel take over their care. It is said that nursing and midwifery outcomes are always difficult to state because health outcomes are notoriously complex. More recently, there has been more emphasis on outcomes rather than on the process of care, and satisfaction rates, healing rates, recovery rates or even readmission rates may be seen as useful. However, it has been noticed that satisfaction outcomes are so intrinsically related to the quality of the health care process that the need to focus on the process of giving care has been given great importance within the NHS. Clinical governance is the latest idea for quality assurance.

Having looked at the notion of quality assurance and the need for standards, you might like to took at your ward/clinical area standards to see which method of standard setting is being utilised and consider whether it is effective.

Clinical governance

The government defined clinical governance (Department of Health 1998) as

> A framework through which NHS organisations are accountable for continuously improving the quality of their services and safeguarding high standards of care by creating an environment in which excellence in clinical care can flourish.

Bassett (1999) suggests that clinical governance can be best summarised as:

a protective mechanism (umbrella) for both the public and healthcare professionals, ensuring that their hospitals and community trusts are actively developing structures to improve the quality of care in the hope of preventing any recurrence of the Bristol Case 1998.

Scally and Donaldson (1998) identified that clinical governance was to be the main method of improving the quality of patient care in the NHS. They stated that it needed organisation-wide transformation, clinical leadership and positive organisational cultures. They highlighted the need for learning from past failures such as variations in standards of care, particularly with respect to breast and cervical screening programmes. They also noted that poor quality is often detected through complaints, audit, untoward incidents or routine surveillance. They proposed that the need for a more open, participative and shared culture, good leadership and team training and working as well as evidence for good practice would be the key to success. Lilley (1999), as the Director of the Clinical Governance Research and Development Unit at the University of Leicester, concurs and suggests that clinical governance:

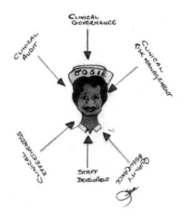

- is everyone's business
- involves patients and service users
- ignores departmental and service boundaries and works across them
- involves everyone in developing their professional capabilities
- is continuous and evolving in its quest for improvement
- is about finding out what works best and doing it every time
- is based on evidence
- is transparent and open.

He highlights the responsibilities of Trusts and primary care groups:

- to establish leadership, accountability and working arrangements
- to carry out quality assessments
- to formulate action plans
- to clarify reporting arrangements.

This means that all practitioners will need to accept responsibility for developing and maintaining standards of care within the local service. Ultimately health care needs to be evidence-based and professionals need to identify the rationale for treatment and care being effective as well as efficient. Crinson (1999) notes five key components for a system of clinical governance:

1. Clinical audit.
2. Clinical effectiveness.
3. Clinical risk management.
4. Quality assurance.
5. Staff development.

These factors will now be considered in turn.

Clinical audit

Dunitz (1995) identifies that audit as a measuring, evaluation or study process, which should improve the medical care that the patient receives. There have been many attempts to do more than set standards. The idea of measuring quality implies that there will be some benchmark of quality acceptability. BS 5750 or the ISO 9000 have been examples of awards (or reaching a certain quality benchmark) in organisations but are often quite mechanistic. Monitoring quality is often linked with the terms 'audit' or 'evaluation'. Morgan and Everitt (1990) offer the following definitions:

- *Monitoring*: The continuous or regularly repeated observations or measurements of important parts of the service structure process output or outcome.
- *Audit*: A discrete activity composing a detailed periodic review of part or whole of a service or a procedure. In audit there is an explicit search for improvement as with correction: this means that the importance of an audit extends beyond monitoring into service development.
- *Evaluation*: Refers to the judgements made on information arising from a monitoring system.

Various national nursing audit tools have been developed in the past, e.g. Monitor, Qualpacs. Difficulty has arisen with a need to modify these tools to suit each unique care environment. There has also been a need to work within multi-disciplinary team audits (clinical audit) now that there are tighter working arrangements and contracting brought about by health legislation. These audits focus now on the patient's experiences rather than the various individual services.

Clinical effectiveness

This is about whether health care interventions achieved the required outcome. Research is needed to identify what those outcomes may be. For instance, you may question the effectiveness of analgesia in pain control. The use of patient-controlled analgesia (PCA) as opposed to conventional prescription and administration may pose specific questions about whether some pain is better controlled using alternative methods.

Discuss with a colleague a recent incident where you have questioned the effectiveness of an intervention or treatment.

It has to be said that there are many questions about health care interventions where even the research is ambiguous. However, Muir Gray (1996) points to key questions about the use of research as evidence for health care. These are related to the relevance of the research, the range of outcomes and effects, generalisability, and whether any intervention does more harm than good. This must be taken in the context of his traditional science background and may not always fit with the nature of nursing and midwifery research, which shows that effective care is often unmeasurable.

Clinical risk management

In a health service attempting to minimise errors and complaints, risk management is an important aspect of forward thinking. Lilley and Lambden (1999) state that there are three aims to risk management that can broadly be seen as follows:

1. Reducing or eliminating the harm to the patient.
2. Dealing with affected patient and supporting clinical staff.
3. Safeguarding the organisational assets.

In terms of a risk assessment for moving and handling, you will see the importance of these aims for patients who are not able to move themselves easily. If every bed in hospital had a slip sheet, maybe more nurses would use them and avoid discomfort/injury to the patient, prevent back injury and reduce high absenteeism and even litigation for the Trusts.

Lilley and Lambden also identified the four principles of risk management:

1. Risk identification.
2. Risk analysis.
3. Risk control.
4. Risk cost.

Try to remember these points when you assess a patient's moving and handling needs.

At a deeper level, risk management involves the ability of all staff to report adverse problems and events without fear of being made a personal scapegoat. This will require courage and more positive support of 'whistleblowing'.

Quality assurance

The ability of the health service to assure quality is an important means to building the confidence of the public but must be taken in the light of what staff feel are important standards. The use of critical care pathways is one example of what patients/clients will expect and what commissioners will expect to build into contracts. Look back at the example of a critical care pathway in Chapter 2 (Figure 2.9). While this is only an example of how quality might be assured, it is also a method of establishing an evaluative process which is what quality assurance, clinical audit and clinical governance is really all about.

Staff development

Ultimately quality relies on well-trained and critical practitioners who are well motivated and enthusiastic to improve care continuously. Clinical governance therefore relies on professional regulation and lifelong learning (see Chapter 12). The importance of PREP requirements is essential but hardly an optimum development framework, with only five days over three years. In a regularly changing health service this is inadequate to provide the quality required. The question of who funds staff development is also an important issue as ultimately the health service clinical governance theme is underpinned by this development.

Conclusion

The main emphasis of this chapter has been to examine the concepts of quality and attempt to relate them to nursing, midwifery and health visiting practice. There are many classical texts related to these concepts but here we have attempted to demonstrate the ways in which the well-recognised texts affect the delivery of health care and the practice of nursing, midwifery or health visiting. Having examined the concepts of quality, we went on to look at the impetuses of the quality movement within the health service together wth the government White Papers, from here moving on to total quality management. Discussion of 'a first class service' followed, looking at the lines of responsibility and quality monitoring activities needing to be undertaken in order to ensure a firm 'quality' delivery of care in whatever arena. The latest 'buzzwords' associated with the quest for excellence in health care delivery include clinical governance, clinical audit, clinical effectiveness, clinical risk management and quality assurance. Finally, we discussed the impact that quality assurance will have on the practice of nursing, midwifery and health visiting in relation to PREP and the requirement to update clinically on a three-yearly basis. These were discussed in turn but clearly wider reading around the issues will assist in your understanding. This chapter will have helped you to consider how the above concepts can be applied within the caring environment.

Summary of key points

This chapter has examined the following areas.

- **Concept of quality:** The British Standards Institute defines quality as 'the totality of features and characteristics of a product or service that bears on its ability to satisfy stated or applied needs'. Nurses, midwives and health visitors may be constrained by government expenditure on health care as a proportion of the GNP together with the four central features related to quality highlighted by WHO (1983).

- **Quality movement in the NHS:** The Patient's Charter (1992), the Health Act 1999, NICE and CHI were all discussed here while examining the impact of monitoring quality in the workplace.

- **TQM:** Highlighted the philosophy related to customer satisfaction.

- **A first-class health service:** Highlighted the Department of Health's policy of 1998 and the need for standard statements which will mean that care can be measured for its effectiveness.

- **Clinical governance:** Is an umbrella term used in order to ensure that hospitals and community Trusts are actively developing structures to improve the quality of care delivery.

- **Clinical audit:** Is a measuring tool in order to evaluate the quality of care delivery.

- **Clinical risk management:** Is an element that affects all work and life practices. One must always assess the risks involved when one carries out a procedure in order to ensure that neither you nor the patient is incurring any unnecessary risk.

References

Bassett C (ed.) (1999) *Clinical Supervision: A Guide for Implementation*, Nursing Times Books

Crinson I (1999) Clinical governance: the new NHS, new responsibilities, *British Journal of Nursing* **8** (7), 449–53

Deming W Edwards (1986) *Out of the Crisis*, Cambridge University Press

Department of Health (1998) *A First Class Service: Quality in the New NHS*, Department of Health

Department of Health (1991) *The Patient's Charter*, HMSO

Donabedian A (1966) Evaluating the quality of medical care, *Millbank Memorial Fund Quarterly*, **44**, 166–206

Drucker P (1967) The effective executive, in Flanagan H, and Spurgeon P (1996) *Public Sector Managerial Effectiveness*, Open University Press

Drummond H (1992) *The Quality Movement*, Kogan Page

Dunitz M (1995) *Clinical Audit*, Martin Dunitz Ltd

Garbett R (1998) Clinical governance? *Nursing Times Learning Curve* **2** (7), 15

Keighley T (1989) Developments in Quality Assurance, *Senior Nurse* **9**, 7 – 10

Kitson A (1988) in WMHA (1990) *Quality and Standard Setting Workshop*, Directorate of Nursing and Quality

Lilley R (1999) *Making Sense of Clinical Governance*, Radcliffe Medical Press

Lilley R and Lambden P (1999) *Making Sense of Risk Management: A Workbook for Primary Care*, Radcliffe Medical Press

Maxwell R J (1984) Quality assurance in health, *BMJ*, **288** 1470–72

Morgan J and Everitt T (1990) *Introducing Quality Management: A Training Manual*, SE Staffordshire HA/Birmingham University

Muir Gray J A (1996) *Evidence-based Health Care*, Churchill Livingstone

Øvretveit J (1992) *Health Service Quality*, Blackwell Scientific Publications

RCN (1998) *Guidance for Nurses on Clinical Governance*, RCN

Rivett G (1998) *From Cradle to Grave: Fifty Years of the NHS*, King's Fund

Scally G and Donaldson L (1998) Clinical governance and the drive for quality improvement in the new NHS in England, BMJ, **317**, 61–5

World Health Organization (1983) *The Principles of Quality Assurance*, WHO 1260–1271 (Report on a WHO meeting)

Further reading

Department of Health (1992) *Minding the Quality: Consultation Document*, Audit Commission

Donabedian A (1986) Criteria and standards for quality assessment and monitoring, *Quality Review Bulletin*, **2**(3), 99–100

Gould T and Merrett H (1992) *Introducing Quality Assurance into the NHS*, Macmillan

Kemp N and Richardson (1990) *Quality Assurance in Nursing Practice*, Butterworth Heinemann

Koch T (1992) A review of nursing quality assurance, *Journal of Advanced Nursing*, **17**, 785–794

NHSME (1993) *The Quality Journey*, Health Publications Unit

NHSE (1998) *Clinical Effectiveness*, NT/NHSE

Redfern S J and Norman I J (1990) Measuring the quality of nursing care: a consideration of different approaches, *Journal of Advanced Nursing* **15**, 1260–1271 RCN (1988) The Dynamic Standard Setting System, Standards of Care Project, RCN

Sale D (1990) *Quality Assurance*, Macmillan

Young K (1994) An evaluative study of a community health service development, *Journal of Advanced Nursing*, **19**, 58 – 65

11

Resourcing the service

By the end of this chapter you will have had the opportunity to:

- recognise the importance of resource management as a nursing activity
- be able to identify the components of resource management in terms of human resource management and non-human resource management
- be able to consider the allocation of resources in health care and nursing at a national and local level
- discuss the importance of effective recruitment, retention and induction of new staff
- recognise the importance of equal opportunities processes
- describe the appraisal process
- demonstrate an awareness of the budget process
- examine the budget setting and cost containment process
- examine the contracting process.

Introduction

Resources are vital to any organisation but for the health service resources are limited by the overall health budget set by the government. Nurses, midwives and health visitors are at the cutting edge of managing resources and, as the biggest group of employees in the NHS, they are one of the most important resources within the whole service itself. The NHS is noted as being one of the largest employers in Europe so it is important that 'people management' is taken seriously. People management is often referred to as human resource management (HRM) which reflects its importance alongside other areas such as financial management or marketing management. An important feature of HRM is the support and control systems in place in relation to the overall efficiency and effectiveness of its people. Support systems give employees *enabling structures* in order to carry out their work to the best of their ability. Control systems complete the management cycle and are concerned with *gauging the achievement* of the organisational objectives and implementing the support systems, which improve organisational performance. Financial management is also related to HRM as people cost money but this is a much broader activity in the health service. Nurses, midwives and health visitors have had to become more aware of the cost of treatment and care in order to improve care quality and become more efficient and effective. For example, the patient or client who is assessed by several people on admission to hospital may find that it is tiring and they and their family see the use of various people asking the same questions as incompetent practice. It also has financial implications when health care professionals are in short supply. This chapter will examine resource management in the light of recruitment, retention and quality people management. Financial management will also be discussed in relation to nursing, midwifery and health visiting control. There is a plethora of information, with whole books and degree programmes written about these elements, so we will be content with examining how resource management may influence the delivery of the health service and demonstrate how it impacts on care provision.

Human resource management

Human resource and personnel management may be seen as the same thing in small organisations and indeed may often be seen as part of one person's role, which may even be tied in with the nursing function. In larger organisations, HRM may be divided up into many different departments such as personnel, training and development and health and safety. Whatever the situation, there is a need to have suitably qualified people, responsible for getting the right people for the job, training, motivating and rewarding staff as well as complying with the laws related to employment. When a newly-qualified nurse or midwife applies for their first job, they do not always realise the role and responsibilities of the personnel or HRM department and do not always recognise the whole range of services open to them.

HRM involves the following characteristics:

- Proactive strategic 'people planning'.
- Employees viewed as subjects with potential for growth and development.
- Management and non-management have a common interest in the success of the organisation.

HRM has a broad range of 'people' interests. These could be categorised into *getting the right people, training, developing and nurturing the right people, and recognising and evaluating the performance of the people in the organisation.* In chronological order, for staff this is about the following processes within a health organisation:

- recruitment and selection
- induction
- health and safety
- appraisal and performance
- training and development
- employee welfare
- disciplinary and grievance
- outplacement.

Getting the right people

The health service requires a whole range of medical, nursing and therapy staff as well as supporting structures to manage and administer their work. It is important that the right qualified and trained people are brought into the service to provide quality health care. In order to acquire the right people, the following plan shows how the overall resource process may appear:

- Trust corporate plan
- staff planning
- job analysis
- job description
- person specification
- recruitment
- interviewing
- selection
- job evaluation.

- Were you aware of this range of activities behind HRM?
- Write down what you think a person specification is.

A 'person specification' identifies the essential and desirable qualities needed for a post (see Table 11.1 for Staff Nurse example). HRM helps organisations and staff to 'fit' together. Job descriptions and person specifications will be covered in Chapter 12. In terms of nursing, midwifery and health visiting posts, these are seen within the context of staffing levels within a whole Trust. *Making a Difference* (Department of Health, 1999) highlighted the recent problems with recruitment and retention of staff which is compounded by the fact there is increased demand for health care and increased expectations of quality care. It was therefore suggested that steps should be taken to increase recruitment through a more flexible entry to nurse education together with greater flexibility in the delivery of courses, i.e. part-time routes.

Table 11.1 Example of person specification

	Essential	Desirable
Physical	● Healthy	
Education/qualifications	● Professional qualification ● Educated to diploma level	● Working towards degree in nursing
Experience nurse		● At least one year at staff level
Aptitudes	● Proven organisational ability ● Able to problem solve	
Interpersonal skills	● Good communication skills (oral and written) ● Ability to work on own while contributing as a team member	
Other requirements	● Must be able to work 12-hour shifts, nights and weekends as required	

Skill mix

Skill mix within the health service has been seen as an important feature and has recently been recognised within the document *A Health Service for All Talents* (Department of Health 2000). Corporate Trust plans involve matching the complexity of skills mix of multi-professionals to the complexity of patient needs for which they have been commissioned. Nerssling defined skill mix as:

> the balance between untrained and trained, qualified and unqualified and supervisory and operative staff within a service area as well as between different staff groups... . Optimum skill mix is achieved when the desired standard of service is provided at the minimum cost, which is consistent with the efficient deployment of trained, qualified and supervisory personnel and the maximisation of contributions from all staff members. It will ensure the best possible use of scarce professional skills to maximise the service to clients (Nerssling 1990, cited by Clark and Copcutt 1997, p. 197)

● Think back on a recent clinical placement and think about the nurses, midwives or health visitors who worked in the area. Identify the names and grade of staff and the skills and contributions they each made to the everyday running of the area
● What issues do you think are raised from skill mix?

You may think about the activities of staff in terms of day-to-day patient/client care: the longer-term activities such as setting of standards, guidelines and protocols, the teaching and development of staff, the types of work that some staff do and others do not, the management, the leadership and even who does and who does not do *the paperwork*! Another point may be that the grade of staff does not necessarily equate to a particular skill or competency. Two E grades in the same unit may have totally different skills (e.g. interpersonal, practical). Clinical managers need to examine the total skill mix within a team by looking at the requirements of the unit, department, ward or team in relation to what is known as the 'establishment'. The establishment figure is a list of the type of staff in terms of their grade or skill together with the number of staff, in whole-time equivalents, that would meet the needs of the patients, clinicians and nurses, within financial constraints. There is often a compromise between the desired and the practical. Establishments were based on an historical formula that allowed for staffing ratios for particular speciality beds and an allowance for annual leave and sickness, which is made up of whole-time equivalents (WTEs) of various grades of staff, qualified and unqualified. The WTE

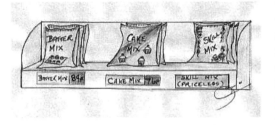

should ideally be determined through a complicated equation which takes into account category of care, turnover rate, length of care episode and dependency. Another reality is that most health care is delivered over a 24-hour period which means that annual salaries are set for day periods only. Evenings, weekends and nights incur 'special duty' payments to staff; other variables will be related to the grades of staff required during these more expensive times of care, thus impacting on the overall budget. In an ideal world, the establishment should be calculated not only at the beginning of a service but on a five-yearly basis in order to ensure that the human resources required to offer a quality service are maintained. However, there is often no scientific calculation applied and the establishment is set within the context of history or due to political pressure. The supply and demand of staff does not always match across the whole health service and where there is great pressure on health services, supply of staff often poses many difficulties, so compounding the pressure on quality services. Understanding the way in which service provision requirements are calculated may make working within the organisation a more satisfying experience.

What do you think affects the recruitment and retention of health service staff?

There are two main factors affecting the supply of staff in the health service:

1. Internal factors.
2. External factors.

Internal factors are those over which employers have some direct influence and include such things as pay, status, perceptions of management style, job satisfaction, career developments and training, and employment conditions. By contrast, *external factors* are those over which the employer has very little control, e.g. total number of employable people; demographic changes; social trends; mobility; economy; cultural attitudes and competition for staff. There are also health service policies related to recruitment, retention, return, deployment and wastage. Together with these policies other factors affecting recruitment need to be considered, such as the decline in school leavers, local levels of unemployment and local competition for employees. Efficient utilisation of resources including staffing has become an increasingly important issue within health care. Nurses make up the largest proportion of NHS staff (estimated to be about 25 per cent) and ultimately consume a large proportion of the NHS budget. The mix of skills or grades over the years has been affected by the following:

- demography
- lack of staff in high tech areas
- P2K
- strategy for nursing
- contracting and commissioning for the services
- resource management focus
- competition under the internal market
- emphasis on quality of care
- re-grading of nurses in 1988.

Recruitment, selection and equal opportunities

Recruitment of staff is now seen in terms of recruiting staff:

- into student places
- straight into positions within clinical care.

This means that the education provider and the health service need to work in partnership to plan appropriate quality curricula, commission numbers required, set criteria for applications and jointly get involved with the process of recruitment and selection. Medical and non-medical education policies exist for the whole of the NHS.

As we move towards the recognition that certain groups in society have been discriminated against in the job market, the importance of equal opportunities for positions and career prospects is an important issue in HRM. The following legislation affects recruitment and selection at all stages:

- Sex Discrimination Act 1975
- Race Relations Act 1976
- Equal Pay Act 1970
- Disabled Persons Act 1944, 1997
- Rehabilitation of Offenders Act 1974
- The Employment Relations Act 1999 (maternity and paternity rights).

As a health care student you may have been aware of some of these issues on application forms that you filled in. The student groups are very different to what they were years ago. There are now greater numbers of men and older applicants entering the caring professions. Indeed, there are now more women entering medicine than there were years ago. Consider the average age of your student group in comparison with the average age of students ten years ago. You may need to ask some of the trained staff in your clinical areas what their student groups were like. You will probably have found that ten years ago the average age of student nurses, midwives and health visitors was somewhat younger than now. This may be directly linked to social trends and the increased number of mature applicants for training. In examining such documents as *Making a Difference* (Department of Health 1999) and *Fitness for Practice* (UKCC 1999), there is a clear indication that the government feels it is necessary to widen the entry gate in order to attract potential students and to attract trained nurses and midwives back into practice. These actions will assist in the recruitment and selection of students into the system. What then of trained staff? The increase in the provision of 'return to practice' courses and subsequent support within clinical areas will enhance patient care. Recruitment should be a planned and systematic event because if you do not know who you are looking for, it is difficult to know when you have found them. It is therefore necessary to have job descriptions and person specifications when embarking on the hunt for suitable personnel. Resource planning may involve filling vacant posts but may also be about creating new posts for new services. HRM in the health service therefore needs to consider recruitment in the light of the following:

- minimum and maximum skill levels
- minimum and maximum staff numbers
- procedures for unplanned absences
- use of pool, bank and agency staff
- record keeping and information systems
- lengths of shifts
- shift pattern.

Training, developing and nurturing

Once an organisation has recruited the right people to deliver quality health care, it is important that managers make sure they settle into the new position and have the ability to 'grow' within the organisation.

Why do you think this is important in the health service?

If you are not helped to settle into the job you would start to become dissatisfied with it, which would ultimately affect the quality of service that you provided to patients, relatives and staff within the organisation. The first stage of joining a new organisation is one of the most stressful times. It is difficult to find your way round the clinical area, get to know all the faces in the workplace and understand what their various roles are. There are new ways of working and the onus is put on you to know these. This is also the most likely time for any health and safety incident to occur due to lack of knowledge and equipment found within the area. This first period of work is known as the induction and orientation period.

Can you remember the type of start you had at university when you began your course? What topics were relevant on the first few days?

You might have been shown around buildings and facilities such as libraries and computer suites as well as being introduced to key people, and you will probably have been given mountains of paperwork to read. You should also have been given an induction in every clinical area you went to, and fire systems and health and safety equipment should have been a top priority. Quite overwhelming, when you look back. Similar feelings occur during final stages of work, i.e. retirement or redundancy, when you might wonder how you are going to cope in the future.

HRM and your own line managers should be concerned that when you start work you have a similar orientation and induction. They will want you to settle into the clinical area with the help of a mentor/preceptor to guide you through the first few weeks. You will also need to know about the whole organisation as well, in terms of how the wages are paid, what services are available to you and how you can get to know about the overall policies of the organisation. You will also need to know what courses and updates you need to attend over and above your own professional development courses. In the NHS, you will need to attend a fire lecture on an annual basis, for instance. If you attend courses, your managers will expect you to give feedback on these and HRM departments will also send out evaluative question-naires. This is all linked to the idea of motivation and the key theories about the quality of working life, which allows staff to feel that they are considered to be of worth and value within a caring work environment.

Appraisal, grievance and disciplinary procedures

Staff development and appraisal schemes are prevalent in today's society. They assist you in reaching your aims by allowing you to reflect upon what you have achieved over the previous year before looking ahead to the coming year and what your aspirations are for that time. It is commonly felt that, through this method of evaluating performance, employees will feel empow-ered to progress their career and gain 'job satisfaction'. In many areas individual performance review (IPR) is linked to the appraisal of clinical skills through clinical supervision and will then be linked to the Trust's overall business plan in terms of commissioning for continuing or in-service educa-tion. Bishop (1998) suggests that the basic format uses the ENB 10 Key Characteristics to provide a benchmark for assessment. As benchmarking in nursing becomes more prevalent, it will be those new benchmarks that will be linked to IPR. Nurses, midwives and health visitors will evaluate their own competence against the statements and agree, through discussion with their line manager, the perceived accuracy of that evaluation. Following the agreement, the discussion will go on to highlight the needs of the individual for the coming year, which will feed into the planning for the provision of courses/training. There are other models that could be utilised in this situa-tion (hierarchical or collegial) but the one described would normally be the model of choice. This is all completed under the umbrella of clinical supervi-sion and as such is seen as a method to encourage and maintain high standards of care, not only for the patient but also for the member of staff and thus staff retention is improved. However, when employer or employee standards are not maintained or deviations from the accepted norm occurs, grievance or disciplinary procedures may be activated.

Employee grievance procedures will be in place within any Trust and typi-cally they will have four stages:

1. Employee talks informally with the line manager as soon as possible after the event.
2. If response to Stage 1 is not satisfactory, then a written appeal may be submitted within ten days of the incident.
3. The employee, union representative, grievance chairperson, HR director and nursing manager will meet for discussions.
4. Arbitration is invoked if there are no solutions to the problem.

It is useful to remember some key behaviour highlighted by Trotta (1976) when involved with hearing a grievance:

1. Put the grievant at ease and let them have their say. Do not interrupt or disagree.
2. Listen openly and carefully. Search for what the employee is trying to say. Take notes.
3. Discuss the problems calmly and with an open mind. Avoid arguments, avoid antagonism and the urge to win. Negotiate.
4. Get the story straight. Get all the facts. Ask logical questions to clarify doubtful points. Distinguish fact from opinion.
5. Consider the grievant's viewpoint. Do not assume s/he is automatically wrong.
6. Avoid snap judgements. Do not jump to conclusions. Be willing to admit mistakes.
7. Make an equitable decision, then give it to the grievant promptly. Do not pass the buck.

Together with this, most managers will have to discipline employees at some time in their careers, i.e. when a rule/regulation or policy has been disregarded. The primary function of discipline, however, is not to punish the guilty party but to teach new skills and encourage that person and others to behave appropriately in the future (Sullivan and Decker 1997). When faced with a matter that requires some form of discipline there is always a policy that will give the manager step-by-step guidance related to how to act. It is also useful to remain in contact with the Human Resource Department to take any advice required about the situation, i.e. before the manager takes any action it must be checked with the department to ensure that no employment law is being contravened. Sullivan and Decker further suggest that in order to ensure fairness, the rules and regulations should be communicated and a system of progressive penalties set up, preferably in writing. Together with this, an appeals process will be built into the system should the guilty party be dissatisfied with the outcome of the hearing.

Financial resource management

Although people are the main backbone of the health service, financial aspects are also a concern to be managed. There is a need today to try to understand the expenses and costs within health care and the need to be more cost aware within professional practice.

HRM and managing staff are therefore obviously linked to a budget and are seen within the realm of financial resource management in the health service. Financial resource management involves the understanding and use of a budget.

Think back to the recent clinical placement where you had identified the names and grade of staff and the skills and contributions they each made to the everyday running of the area.

- Could you identify the approximate annual cost of this workforce within this one small area of the health service?
- What else would you need to help with the calculation?

You would need to identify the variables related to:

- the average salary of each particular grade
- whether some people were full time or need paying pro rata
- the special duty payment cost
- cost of drugs
- cost per day of keeping someone in hospital.

This makes the calculation more complex, don't you think? There are other costs as well which include bank or agency cover for sickness holiday, study leave or maternity leave.

Hammond (1991) defines a budget as 'a statement of the financial position of a person, business or other organisation for a future period of time based on estimates of expenditure and proposals for financing them'. But Taylor (1992) simply says that a budget is an *agreed* plan about the *future operations* of an organisation expressed in *quantitative* terms'. This latter definition shows that budgeting is more about planning, agreeing and managing resources. Taylor, as a public sector accountant, goes on to say that all organisations use budgets to plan and control their operations; the technique of budgeting has an important place in the management process. It is the plan that expresses the intentions as agreed through the management process. The plan is not written in 'tablets of stone' but is the agreed working position; it also indicates the future decisions and includes more than just the financial constraints. The quantitative terms will provide a more definitive statement, e.g. five additional nurses will be recruited in September.

Patient/client dependency

There has been much work done on patient/client dependency levels and the need for specific skills and professional judgement and activity for particular dependencies. For example, Freeman, *et al.* (1999) identified four categories of dependency within district nursing:

1. Long term/ palliative.
2. Rehabilitative care.
3. Administration of prescribed/requested treatments.
4. Educative/supportive/advice care.

Within each of these categories, they aligned a time range which could then be costed and the financial cost of the service could then be measured. There is now a move towards staffing to a budget rather than a historical establishment. This allows for more flexibility but potentially raises concern for attracting and recruiting the right skills in the care environment. Where staff may find difficulty recruiting qualified staff, they can make decisions to dilute the qualified with unqualified or even various grades. Qualified staff may start taking on new skills required within a setting and some of these skills may even be seen historically within the realm of other professional groups. Lifelong career structures and multi-skilling are now part of the flexible approach that the government wishes to pursue. It also forms a basis for contemporary controversial issues that need professional airing. The peaks and troughs of expected workload affect the work rota within clinical areas and the quality of care that can be delivered.

Costs and cost centres

A budget is normally set for each 'cost centre' within a Trust or health service facility. A cost centre refers to a particular service unit, directorate or department, which holds its own budget. Each centre is then accountable to the next unit up in the hierarchy of the Trust or facility. Each cost centre may be aware of various budgets, depending on the type of costs. There are two main categories of costs:

1. *Fixed costs* are the average costs that are not related to the numbers of patients or clients demanding the service, e.g. lighting, heating, etc.
2. *Variable costs* are the average costs that are affected by the supply and demand for the service, e.g. cost of running an ultrasound service.

The difference between these two types of costs has implications for the efficiency of a service and the 'value for money' requirement within the contracting and commissioning of health care services.

The typical breakdown of costs in a ward or clinical area may be as follows:

- staff costs, e.g. salaries
- salary related, e.g. National Insurance and superannuation employer contributions
- consumables, e.g. dressings, drugs, linen, stationery
- overheads, e.g. building, car parking, maintenance
- services, e.g. laundry, domestic, telephone.

Jot down why you think it is important for nurses, midwives and health visitors to be aware of this type of financial resource management and budgeting?

In order to be accountable for our professional actions and to demonstrate value for money we must be aware of methods of effective financial management. Sullivan and Decker (1997) suggest that because nursing activities account for as much as 50 per cent of an organisation's total expenditure, nurse managers need to be proficient at constructing a budget and we also need to play our part in keeping within that projected sum.

Purpose of budgeting

Budgeting in health care involves accounting for the service in financial terms to the taxpayers and government. Taylor (1992) suggested that the budget reflected a process:

- to decide priorities
- to secure resources
- to communicate, coordinate and control activities
- to review performance.

These all appear very important criteria within a finite resource allocation for health in this country. All Trusts are required to set an annual budget and in general this annual budget is seen as a quantitative statement, usually in monetary terms, of the organisation's expectations over the year in order to manage financial performance. Table 11.2 shows six different categories into which a budget may be divided.

Table 11.2 Key budgetary terms

Zero-based budget	A budget approach that assumes that a base for projecting next year's budget is zero. Managers are required to justify every pound in terms of service delivery. This is normally used for brand new units or services.
Fixed budget	Here the amounts are set irrespective of changes that occur during the year but are based on activity from the previous year plus a determined amount extra based on inflation and proposed pay awards. This is sometimes known as a 'historical budget'.
Variable budget	This type of budget allows for adjustments during the year and may also be called 'activity based'. The management accountant needs to know what is happening in a given area at all times.
Operating budget	This is a statement of expected revenues and expenses for the forthcoming year.
Fiscal year	A specific twelve-month period when operational and financial performance is measured.
Revenue budget	A projection of expected income for the budget period based on volume and mix of patients together with the charge rates and discounts that may be given.

- Think of your own personal finances.
- How would you go about working out how much you spent last month?

Some people record all their expenditure by retaining their receipts, completing cheque stubs and keeping records in computer programs, while others wait for the bank manager to inform them when they are not doing too well! Whichever method you adopt, you are aware that an account of your action/expenditure has to be made. This is also vital to an organisation such as the NHS which deals in many millions of pounds of expenditure per year.

However the budget is set, it is the responsibility of the budget holder to remain within the parameters of that budget. For a clinical manager, this is a constant battle between containing spending, maintaining quality standards and fulfilling the demand for the service. One way of doing this is by spending money only on agreed plans and forgoing starting new services without feasibility studies, and agreeing decisions to cost out the consequences. Another is to keep staffing levels within funded establishment. The nominated budget holder holds the ultimate budget responsibility but may be able to delegate to others who can use an agreed budget code. A good information system is therefore vital to support the financial resource accounting required.

Budgeting management skills

Some financial skills are required to understand and manage financial information. Long-term and short-term planning and control are required.

Think about how you control your own stock cupboard at home.

At the start of the month you might not think about the cost required to live, but as you get to the stage when there is 'too much month and not enough money' you might give greater thought to how to manage. You see advertisements on television these days inviting you to place so much of your cash into an account each month in order to pay your bills as they arise, leaving you with money in your normal account that is for you to spend as you will. This is a type of budgetary management. How do Trusts or clinical areas manage their budget when the money is running short? Options may include the following:

- delay spending on any one-off items until the next financial year, e.g. postpone buying replacement equipment.
- communicate the current financial position to staff and ask for their cooperation in making economies

- review who is authorised to charge to your budget and what their spending limits are
- tighten the procedures for issuing and using consumable items
- undertake a 'value for money' exercise on non-pay expenditure by reviewing the use of consumables and possible wastage
- review unsociable hours worked and the use of overtime
- review working rotas of staff
- review staff skill mix
- freeze recruitment.

These all hold ethical and moral questions for the budget holder and are decisions that may not be taken lightly. However, public services need to budget in the same way as individuals, and need to plan expenditure on the basis of expected income. There are some basic financial management skills that you may wish to consider for your future development:

- *Interpretation:* Understanding financial reports; seeing the broad picture.
- *Forecasting:* Historical information is not useful unless it can give guidance for the future. Forecasting skills allow the budget holder to understand the current position in order to take action.
- *Variance analysis:* Is the skill of analysing the difference between what was expected (budget) and the real expenditure. There is a need to know all possible influences, e.g. underspends (favourable/negative variances) and overspends (unfavourable/positive variables).

Think about why we need to be able to gain these skills within our own professional development. Write down two points.

It could be said that there is a need to understand that pay issues can be affected if there are more/fewer staff in post than funded establishment, or if there is a different skill mix in post than funded, this will have a knock-on effect. Together with this, if there was a miscalculation of the number of unsociable hours worked at night and weekends than budgeted for, or staff in post have different points on a salary scale to those budgeted for, again this would need investigation. There may be other things going on in the area such as changes in working practice, irregular purchasing, changes in workload or high sickness levels. On a political note, if we do not manage and account for our own professional budget, another department may start making decisions for us which may compromise our standards of care.

Financial resource management and the balance sheet

The balance sheet, as a statement of the financial position of an organisation at a given date, is often perceived as 'the budget account'. It shows the organisation's resources on that date in terms of what it owns and what it owes, i.e. assets and liabilities. The assets and liabilities should balance. Public or private investors are shareholders/stakeholders and have provided money and resources for health investment. It is important to the interested parties that the budget should balance favourably.

> Make an effort to access your local Trust's annual report in the Trust or university library. You should note the layout of the accounting section. Discover the annual budget figure and the percentage of that which covers staff costs.

Conclusion

This chapter has examined a variety of resource strategies that might be used within the health service in order to ensure the delivery of 'quality' care. The two elements particularly examined were human resource management and financial management. HRM is a vital part of the organisation if it is proactive, views employees as subjects with potential growth and development and shares a common interest in the success of the organisation. HRM is about getting the right people, then training, developing and nurturing the right people. Once the HRM department has assisted in the employment of the correct people, it then becomes the responsibility of the ward or department manager to ensure that the skill mix is appropriate for each shift, again to ensure that a quality service is delivered. While recruitment may be a major role of the HRM department, there are a variety of government Acts that need to be taken into account, e.g. the Sex Discrimination Act (1975) and the Race Relations Act (1976), to name but two. Following employment there is a need for policies, protocols and procedures within certain situations, for example:

- appraisal – which can be linked to professional development and even promotion
- grievance – where an employee is able to highlight a problem that needs to be addressed;
- disciplinary – when a rule/regulation has been disregarded.

Financial resource management highlights the need for managers to understand and use a budget effectively. Changes in the ways that staffing might be linked to budget rather than 'establishment' was briefly discussed, together with the key budgetary terms and how they may be applied to the clinical environment.

Summary of key points

This chapter has examined the following areas:

- **Human resource management:** Highlighted the many functions of this department which include appointments, training, motivating and rewarding staff and complying with the laws related to employment.

- **Getting the right people:** Described the importance of job descriptions, person specifications, recruitment and interviewing, selection and job evaluation.

- **Skill mix:** Is vital in order to ensure that a high standard of care is delivered safely and effectively.

- **Recruitment, selection and equal opportunities:** Is a major part of ensuring that the right people are employed in the right jobs within the confines of the law, taking into consideration a variety of government Acts.

- **Training, development and nurturing:** Demonstrated the need for employers to 'care' for employees and to ensure that retention of staff is paramount in the smooth running of the organisation.

- **Appraisal, grievance and disciplinary procedures:** Discussed the need for staff development and appraisal in order to establish the need for in-service training and continuing professional development. By evaluating performance, employees will gain job satisfaction. Grievance and disciplinary procedures are also a sign of dealing with problems in a modern society. Years ago employed staff did not identify problematical areas, whereas today policies and procedures are in place to deal with grievance and disciplinary matters.

- **Financial resource management:** Examined ways in which the budget of the health service and clinical areas might be arranged. Effective budgeting is essential to maintain the smooth running of the NHS.

References

Bishop V (ed.) (1998) *Clinical Supervision in Practice: Some Questions and Answers*, Macmillan/NT Research

Clark J and Copcutt L (1997) *Management for Nurses and Health Care Professionals*, Churchill Livingstone

Department of Health (1999) *Making a Difference: Strengthening the Nursing, Midwifery and Health Visiting Contribution to Health and Health Care*, The Stationery Office

Department of Health (2000) *A Health Service for all Talents*, The Stationery Office

Freeman S, Shelley G, Gray M and Ingram B (1999) Measuring services: a district nursing dependency tool, *Nursing Standard*, **13**(47), 39 – 41

Hammond S (1991) *Business Studies*, Longman

Sullivan E J and Decker P J (1997) *Effective Leadership and Management in Nursing*, (4th edn) Addison Wesley

Taylor N (1992) *Budgeting Skills: A Guide for Nurse Managers*, Central Health Studies

Trotta M S (1976) *Handling Grievances: A Guide for Management and Labor*, Bureau of National Affairs

UKCC (1999) *Fitness for Practice* (The Peach Report), UKCC

York A (1995) *Managing for Success: A Human Approach*, Cassell in association with the ISM

Further reading

Armstrong M (1990) *Management Processes and Functions*, Institute of Personnel Management

Bailey D (1996) Budgeting skills, Nursing Standard, **10**(19) 43–6

Davies C (1990) *The Collapse of the Conventional Career: The Future of Work and its Relevance for Post Registration Education in Nursing Midwifery and Health Visiting*, ENB

Gasking T (1991) *How to Master Finance: A No-nonsense Guide to Understanding Business Accounts*, Business Books

Iles V (1997) *Really Managing Health Care*, Open University Press

Leavitt H J (1965) Applied organisational change in industry: structural, technological and humanistic approaches, in Mullins L J (1989) *Management and Organisational Behaviour* (2nd edn) Pitman

Makin P, Cooper C and Cox C (1989) *Managing People at Work*, The British Psychological Society and Routledge

McKenna E (1994) *Business Psychology & Organisational Behaviour: A Students' Handbook*, Lawrence Erlbaum Associates

Mullins L J (1999) *Management and Organisational Behaviour* (5th edn) Pitman

Williams H (1994) *The Essence of Managing People*, Prentice Hall

Part

IV

Conclusion

12

Your next move

By the end of this chapter you will have had the opportunity to:

- consider the way forward in terms of career opportunities
- identify the role of professional health care workers in the context of changing health care services
- recognise the knowledge and skills required for future practice
- identify the opportunities and possibilities for professional practice
- discuss the impact of national and local initiatives
- demonstrate an awareness of the impact of new government legislation.

Introduction

Earlier chapters of this book have examined many aspects of management theory, and this final chapter brings us full circle as we again look at you as an individual: where you are going in your career and how you are going to maintain your registration in the future. Once you have gained your initial qualification your enthusiasm for caring, in whatever field, needs to be nurtured. On registration you are deemed to be competent; clinically knowledgeable; skilled; able to assess, plan, implement and evaluate patient care; able to take charge of the clinical areas; able to handle difficult circumstances; and a host of other things. In reality, however, many newly qualified nurses, midwives and health visitors feel anything but competent or confident to move from student status to qualified status. Kramer (1974) coined the term 'the reality shock' of moving from student status into full professional accountability. Expectations and reality, linked with idealism, commitment, stress and changing behaviour, are noted as elements of the 'shock' and are associated with the socialisation into the new role (Marquis and Huston 2000). If you were to undertake another SWOT analysis (see Chapter 1) it might look very different in the area of greatest threat. We need to examine how to cope with the transition. Following this we will look at career pathways; going on to examine practice in the 'new millennium'; finally we will look at the Post-Registration Education Project (PREP) in terms of how you are going to meet those requirements.

Coping with transition

The biggest factor in coping is probably recognising and coming to terms with role expectations (Chapter 4) and managing change (Chapter 8). Buckenham (1988) conducted a study that suggests that the perceptions of the role of staff nurse differed from first- to third-year students. However, the closer one got to qualification, the greater the importance of management skills seemed to be, even to the extent of detracting from the importance of actual clinical nursing care. So how did this happen? Humphries (1987) found that 84 per cent of newly qualified nurses felt that the increase in administrative responsibility was a major factor. However, around 50 per cent also thought that altered relationships were the greatest challenge. It would appear that with the change in status came the perception that the qualified professional knew everything and their opinions suddenly counted for something. Likewise, patients and relatives may be seen to treat qualified professionals differently from students.

One of the aims of Project 2000, diplomas in higher education and degree courses today is to increase awareness of management theory and practice in order to try to reduce the impact of the administrative workload. This type of education also hopes to give you skills to cope with the transition and expectations. While there may be perceived gaps in clinical expertise, they are quickly rectified because you have the knowledge base on which to anchor practice. It is interesting to note that 'traditionally' trained nurses, midwives and health visitors will suggest that others trained today are less able, practically, to cope with the demands of patient/client care. However, the overall training programmes remain 50 per cent theory to 50 per cent practice – not too dissimilar to the 40 per cent theory and 60 per cent practice of previous years. The 10 per cent increase in theory then enables the nurse, midwife or health visitor to apply a sound knowledge base to practice. It could be said that learning to be a qualified nurse, midwife or health visitor is not unlike learning to drive a car. You only really learn to drive after you have passed your test, otherwise why do we have green 'L' plates? Nobody expects a newly qualified driver to be competent or confident at all aspects of driving, so why should it be so for the newly qualified nurse, midwife or health visitor? It is once you have qualified that you learn to cope on your own.

Learning to cope on your own will gradually occur with the help of your mentor or preceptor. The English National Board for Nursing, Midwifery and Health Visiting (ENB) (1993) advised that every newly qualified nurse, midwife or health visitor would have an identified person (mentor or preceptor) on whom they could rely to assist them during the transition. Hanks (1983) states that a mentor is 'A wise and trusted advisor or guide: a friend whom Odysseus put in charge of his household when he left for Troy. He was the advisor of the young Telemachus' whereas Marquis and Huston (2000) state that a preceptor is 'an experienced nurse who provides emotional support and is a strong clinical role model for the new nurse.' Whatever you call this person, they should be there to help you through the transition in order to effect your change of status in the least stressful way.

Career opportunities: the way forward

It has often been said that, following your training, the world will be your oyster. You and your training will be accepted anywhere in the world. Indeed, Hancock (2000) said 'As a highly skilled professional, you share with people many of the most important times in their life. It's a tremendous privilege and responsibility.' It is impossible to describe a typical nursing, midwifery or health visiting career, but as you qualify you will have the skills that can be developed over a wide range of specialities. Many Trusts now advertise rotational posts for newly qualified nurses in order to assist in the decision making as you consolidate your training. This implements the human relations approach to management which demonstrated the theory behind job rotation. In consolidating your training you will also gain experience of 24-hour care but possibly in a variety of settings.

Hydes-Greenwood and Sargent (2001) suggest that progression in your career path is less likely to be vertical in nature as it was in the past, but those pathways are likely to be diverse in order to assist you in achieving a career plan. Your own career plan needs to be drawn up, as a guide, in order to assist you in overall planning. Table 12.1 gives a potted history of the career pathway of an individual but your planning may take you down a totally different pathway. The questions you might like to ask when considering this exercise are as follows:

- What do I want to do?
- What are my skills?
- What further skills and knowledge do I want to acquire?
- What would I enjoy doing?
- Who and what could help me?

This career path will not be written in 'tablets of stone' but will act as a guide and indicate possible direction, timeframe and ultimate goal. In addition, appraisal or review can act to enhance your overall plan or give indication if a change of direction needs to be considered. It is at this point that you can

Table 12.1 Career path – Trace Element

1996–1999	Student Nurse
Experienced nursing in different settings. Gynaecology most interesting	
1999–2003	Staff Nurse
Develop skills in Gynaecology Unit. Undertake further study to develop expertise.	
2002	
Undertake Women's Studies degree in order to raise standards of care within the Gynaecology Unit.	
2004	
Sister of Gynaecology Unit.	

negotiate with your manager how your clinical, teaching and managerial needs will be met. This may be through experience, effective preceptorship and further education. However, it may be reasonable to leave approximately twelve to eighteen months following qualification before embarking on further study. During this time you will be busy consolidating your knowledge and gaining further knowledge related to the specific area of practice. You may also be involved in clinical projects, supervision of learners and mentoring junior staff – all roles to come to terms with. Together with this, if you are in a rotational post lasting eighteen months you may be changing clinical areas up to three times – again another element to come to terms with. At the end of this experience it will be time to consider seriously where your future in nursing might lie. Will it be in clinical specialist nursing, research, education or management? Together with all the opportunities to develop practice skills within this country, there are others abroad. However, it must be recognised that the only real qualification currency for working abroad is RN (Adult) or its equivalent (RGN/SRN) as other countries do not have the same training recognition; they may see mental health nursing, learning disabilities nursing and children's nursing as integral parts of a nursing qualification. Information related to this can be obtained free (for RCN members) from the RCN website. Similarly, you might be required to sit the relevant board examinations in order to practise in another country. In the main, people who originate from an English-speaking country seem to seek employment in countries that are also predominantly English speaking unless they have a personal flair for languages (Table 12.2). Also these opportunities are mainly for single people as it is easier for the employer to arrange the necessary paperwork and accommodation.

Table 12.2 Common overseas destinations for qualified nurses

- Australia; New Zealand; Canada; United States of America.
- Middle East – Kingdom of Saudi Arabia; Oman; Bahrain; Kuwait.
- Voluntary Service Overseas (VSO) – Africa; former Soviet Union; South America.
- European Union – Usually for those with language skills

Agency work is another area that will give you the opportunity to experience the delivery of care in a wide variety of settings in a flexible manner (i.e. hours to suit you). Care must be taken when selecting an agency. A variety of questions should be asked in relation to this:

- Is it registered?
- How long has it been operating?
- Is it a member of a professional body?
- What are their office hours?
- What opportunities do you have to contact them outside normal office hours?
- How do they select and place nurses?
- Is the selection process fair and demonstrating equal opportunities?
- Do you have an interview?
- Do they have a staff training policy?
- What rates of pay do they offer?
- Do they have overseas placements?

If you get positive answers to these questions then it would seem that you are on to a good thing. It really all depends on what you are looking for. The opportunities are endless: you just have to determine what you want out of your career.

Applying for your chosen role

Having decided which direction your career is going to take, it may be an opportune moment to consider the application process by addressing the following:

- your letter of enquiry
- your curriculum vitae (CV) and what it will include
- the job description
- the person specification
- the informal visit
- preparing for the interview
- your acceptance of the post.

Your letter of enquiry (Figure 12.1) is almost the most important part of the process as it sets the impression of who you are and what you are about. It should therefore be written legibly or typed (always black ink and white unlined paper) identifying why you wish to apply for a post, where you might have seen any advertisement, and requesting the appropriate application forms. This letter will be kept with the rest of the documents you provide and used to form an overall picture of you. Initially your CV, which accompanies your enquiry letter, will only be one page in length (Figure 12.2) and will allow the prospective employer a brief glimpse of you as a professional person. You will later submit a more in-depth CV which includes reflection on previous practice together with a detailed history of previous posts and attainments (Figure 12.3). In order to get this into some sort of perspective it is often useful to conduct a SWOT analysis (Chapter 1; see also Figure 12.4). This will enable you to identify constraints on performance causing inefficiencies, but also the strengths that you can offer the new post, thus enabling you to present yourself in the best light.

Periodic Table
Space
SP1 2OU
Date

Their address

Dear Mr Mann

I would like to enquire whether you have any vacancies within the gynaecological area of your hospital.

I am a recently qualified Staff Nurse and will be moving into your area during the next two months. I would value the opportunity to visit your hospital and receive any relevant recruitment information

I enclose my CV for your information.

Yours sincerely,

Trace Element

Figure 12.1 Example of letter of enquiry

Now put yourself on the other side of the picture for a moment – in the position of the employer. Prior to the interviews you have to draw up a reasonable short-list by sifting through the presentations and the information you have received. You turn your tired eyes to application no. 45. It is handwritten, your name is misspelt, the qualifications and experience seem to be suitable but the supporting evidence seems to have been written, initially, for another post. Some of the information/reflection has a slightly facetious tone and the punctuation is appalling. Does this application get on the short list? Probably not.

	Trace Element		
	Periodic Table		
	Space		
	SP1 2OU		
	012 3456 7890 (Home)		
	023 4567 8901 (Work)		
	Date of Birth: 21 May 1976		
School	1992	1994	Part-time Replenishment Assistant, Cosmic Shopping Mall
School	1994		Duke of Edinburgh Silver Award
School	1994		A Levels
			English – C
			Geography – C
			General Studies - D
School	1992		English - B
			Mathematics – B
			Science – C
			Geography – C
			Child Development - D
			Information Technology - C
'Gap Year'	1994	1995	Teaching English in Mexico and India
Care Assistant	1995	1996	Caring for the elderly within a Nursing Home
Student Nurse	1996	1999	

Figure 12.2 Example of Curriculum Vitae (CV)

Once the applicant has the person specification (Table 12.3) and the job description (Table 12.4) relating to the specific job, another useful exercise is for them to conduct a job analysis (Figure 12.5). Any unanswered questions can then be identified for use during the informal visit. Informal visits are often a good way of introducing yourself to your prospective employer, but remember that although they are 'informal', decisions can be made about you at the time so do go prepared to present yourself in the best possible light. Similarly, at this time you may walk into the place and think that you do not wish to proceed with the application as it does not feel right. You may of course walk in and think 'this is the place for me'. The same goes for whoever is showing you round – they will make a judgement about whether or not you would 'fit' in the organisation.

Preparing for your interview is a daunting exercise. It is a time of great stress. An interview is essentially a conversation with a specific purpose but within this exercise you have to prove to the prospective employer that you are the best person for the job, and seek out information about the philosophy, business plan and staffing policies of the Trust/employer company. The more you know about the potential employers, the better. On the day of the interview do ensure that you have left plenty of time to get ready and do arrive slightly early so that you have time to calm down and relax. It is useful to know what you are going to be doing for the rest of the day as interview panels will often contact you later to let you know of the outcome. Remember, before you speak you will be seen. The style of dress you choose indicates that you have a grasp on what is acceptable for the Trust/company but do ensure that it is comfortable (new shoes are often not a good idea in case they pinch!).

Front Sheet	Name; qualifications; position applied for
Second Page	Present role responsibilities; aspirations
Consecutive Pages	Present role including reflection on practice (using a model of reflection)
	Education/qualifications Professional qualifications
	Past roles (latest first) including a reflective summary on each
	Professional bodies; Research interests
	Publications; Professional reading;
	Interests
Final Page	Personal biography (address; telephone numbers; date of birth); referees

Figure 12.3 Headings for extended CV

Think about what they might ask you:

- current issues related to nurse, midwife or health visitor training or practice (the editorials of professional journals are a good source of information) and government policies
- why you want this particular job
- what has been your greatest achievement in your career so far
- where you see yourself in five years' time
- why you think you would be good at this particular job.

STRENGTHS	WEAKNESSES
Skills Qualifications Life experiences Professional experiences Personality Self-presentation	Age Gender Skills; experiences; qualifications Time keeping Planning/organising Introverted/extroverted Narrow/broad focused
THREATS	OPPORTUNITIES
Insufficient appropriate skills insufficient appropriate experience Insufficient appropriate knowledge	'Fit' with job description Training Career development New courses New experiences

Figure 12.4 SWOT Analysis for role suitability

Factual information	• What; when; why; where; and how is the job done
Responsibility	• Subordinates • Equipment • Health and safety • Finance/budget
Relationships	• Superiors • Subordinates • Multi-agency • Disciplinary • Clients/patients
Job requirements	• Skills • Experience • Qualifications • Personality • Motivation • Social skills • Past performance
Working conditions	• Physical • Social • Economic

Figure 12.5 Job analysis

Table 12.3 Example of person specification

	Essential	**Desirable**	**Disqualifiers**
Physical	Healthy		More than 30 days' illness in past year
Attainment	First-level registration; diploma	Degree in nursing	
Intelligence	Average intelligence	Able to work independently and undertake projects	
Aptitudes	Articulate	Computer skills	
Interests		Outside activities	
Disposition and attitudes	Reliable; pleasant personality; punctual	Self-discipline; non-smoker	Poor attendance; unable to get on with people
Special circumstances			

Table 12.4 Example of a job description

Job Title	Staff Nurse
Grade	'D' Grade Staff Nurse
Professional Qualification	RN (Adult)
Accountable to	
Reports to	

Job Philosophy:

The post holder is responsible for the assessment of needs and development of programmes of care, and/or the implementation and evaluation of those programmes. The post holder is expected to carry out all relevant forms of care without direct supervision and may be required to demonstrate procedures to, and supervise qualified or unqualified staff.

Responsibility for meeting the UKCC's requirements in line with the Code of Professional Conduct, accountability and other documents issued by the council rests with the practitioner, as does the responsibility for managing resources within span of control, and promoting team-work with personnel of own and other agencies.

1. Professional/Clinical Functions

- Comply with UKCC Code of Professional Conduct.
- Participate in delegated nursing care programmes.
- Administer medication by whatever route, strictly according to Trust policies and complying with the UKCC Administration of Medicines Code and the Controlled Drugs Act.
- Have regard for patients' customs, religious beliefs and doctrines.
- Ensure that reports on patients, both verbal and written, take due regard to confidentiality and that the UKCC Code of Professional Practice relating to confidentiality is adhered to.
- Participate in teaching of patients, relatives/carers, staff or other agencies as required.

2. **Administrative**

● Maintain appropriate liaison with colleagues in the multi-disciplinary team.

● Maintain accurate, relevant, contemporaneous records and reports as required.

● Comply with Trust requirements as regards data collection either written or via use of a light pen.

● Be accountable for the requisitioning and effective use of resources, physical and non-physical within span of control.

● Facilitate a two-way communication channel with managers in conjunction with the DNS/CN and carry out agreed procedures regarding performance review and provision of data for statistical and planning purposes.

● Be aware of and comply with Trust policies including Health and Safety at Work.

3. **Nurse Education**

● Take every reasonable opportunity to maintain and improve professional knowledge and competence.

● Instruct, support and guide staff, ensuring that they are competent in their knowledge of clinical matters and ward management.

● Participate in induction and in-service education programmes for staff.

4. **Personnel**

● Work in a collaborative and cooperative manner with other health care professionals and recognise and respect their particular contribution within the health care team.

NB: This job description is not exhaustive and will be reviewed and amended at regular intervals in the light of developing organisational need and in consultation with the post holder.

During the interview do take time to consider your answer and assemble your thoughts. This will impress the interview panel, and you will then provide a well-constructed answer. At the end of the interview it is usual to be invited to ask any questions. If you have taken up the opportunity of an informal visit then most of your questions will have been answered. Do say if they were covered during the informal visit (this demonstrates the interest you have shown in the job by going out of your way to visit before continuing), but you might enquire about further education and training support. It is also polite to thank the panel for their time and interest while shaking hands. Following the offer of a post you must write and indicate your acceptance or rejection of that post – you never know if you might want to go there in the future, even if you change your mind now.

Practising in the new millennium

At the start of a new century, nursing, midwifery and health visiting face some challenges ahead. *Healthcare Futures 2010* (Welsh Institute for Health and Social Care 1998), commissioned by the UKCC, identified many future changes for the nursing, midwifery and health visiting professions, brought about by the many social, political and economic forces. Importantly this text shows the many unresolved paradoxes within health care.

Interestingly, in terms of the health service there is also uncertainty. The University of Glamorgan (Welsh Institute for Health and Social Care 1998) has proposed three scenario visions for the future of health care:

1. A 'constrained' service based on a collectivist ethos.
2. An expensive service based on a consumer-driven powerbase.
3. A 'safety net' service running alongside private and other provision.

These visions provide us with alternative pictures of a health service in the twenty-first century.

The key trends that the health service will have to address are as follows:

- increased chronic non-communicable diseases, i.e. circulatory, cancer, gastro-intestinal and metabolic diseases
- growing numbers with mental ill health
- obesity caused by over-eating and sedentary occupations
- emerging and resurgent infectious diseases.

There are also growing trends of consumerism which links with the idea that choice is a political ideology and this will challenge the knowledge and powerbase of professionals. The Heathrow Debate paper (Department of Health 1994) emphasised the need for changes within the professions to fit the changing world. It pointed out, however, that there are certain health professional roles that should be kept constant:

- a coordinating function
- a teaching function
- developing and maintaining programmes of care
- technical expertise used directly or indirectly
- concern for the ill as well as those currently well
- a special responsibility for the frail and vulnerable.

During 1999 two important documents were issued: *Making a Difference* (Department of Health 1999a) and *Fitness for Practice* (UKCC 1999). Both of these documents serve to give direction to nursing, midwifery and health visitor education and standards. It is worth while examining them in some detail in order to establish the way forward for nursing, midwifery and health visiting.

Making a Difference

> Making a Difference explains the Government's strategic intentions for Nursing, Midwifery and Health Visiting and its commitment to strengthen and to maximise the nursing, midwifery and health visiting contribution. But this needs to be matched by the personal professional commitment of every nurse, midwife and health visitor. (Moores 1999)

Within this document there are statements that demonstrate the value placed on the contribution of nurses, midwives and health visitors in the delivery of care. The document goes on to identify nine areas (Table 12.5) which will now be addressed and enhanced.

Table 12.5 Making a Difference (1999)

1. New nursing in the new NHS.
2. Recruiting more nurses.
3. Strengthening education and training.
4. Developing a modern career framework.
5. Inproving working lives.
6. Enhancing quality of care.
7. Strengthening leadership.
8. Modernising professional self-regulation.
9. Working in new ways.

New nursing in the new NHS
There is a statement that tells us that the context of care is changing. People are living longer, so the number of elderly people in the population is rising and the demand for care in the community is increasing. Trends in the patterns of disease are changing both nationally and globally. Technology will benefit health care with innovations such as NHS Direct and NHS Net. The expectations that are changing are highlighted in papers such as the following:

- *The New NHS: Modern, Dependable* (1997)
- *The Information for Health: An Information Strategy for the Modern NHS 1998 to 2005* (1998)
- *A First Class Service: Quality in the New NHS* (1998)
- *The New NHS - Working Together: Securing a Quality Workforce for the NHS* (1998)
- *Modernising and Social Services: Promoting Independence, Improving Protection, Raising Standards.* (1998)
- *Modernising Mental Health Services: Safe, Sound and Secure* (1998)

- *Smoking Kills* (1998)
- *Saving Lives: Our Healthier Nation* (1999)
- *Sure Start* (1999)
- *The NHS Plan.*

Each of these are well worth reading. It is recommended that you look at them, particularly the ones specifically related to your proposed practice area.

Recruiting more nurses
Between 1992 and 1994 the number of training places available was reduced by 28 per cent (Department of Health 1999, p. 19) but the tide is turning, with recruitment from schools and further education institutions increasing. Together with this, a national campaign was launched to attract nurses, midwives and health visitors back to the profession through 'return to practice' courses.

Strengthening education and training
There is to be provision of more career opportunities, e.g. from cadet, to nurse, to midwife, to health visitor, or to consultant nurse. Together with this, a Partner's Council will be established to provide a framework for post regis- tration and continuing professional development. Flexible pre-registration programmes with 'step-on/step-off' points and part-time courses leading to initial registration are also features of proposed trends to strengthen education and training.

Developing a modern career framework
The proposed career trajectory depicted in Figure 12.6 describes a career framework where progression is linked to the responsibilities and competen- cies needed to do the job rather than application and interview (although this element will still feature in recruitment and retention).

Improving working lives
NHS-wide standards for implementation of supportive, family-friendly poli- cies; sharing of good practice; provision of practical support; together with nurses, midwives and health visitors will be involved in all decision-making affecting their working lives. It is unclear whether this will be on an individ- ual basis or through representation within a committee structure. Employers are required to tackle discrimination, harassment and violence in the work- place. Quite how this will be implemented is still unclear, as each Trust will have its own policy and procedure.

Enhancing quality of care
This will be attained through the use of clear national standards, clinical gov- ernance, evidence-based practice and a strategy for undertaking research (discussed in Chapter 9). Many Trusts already have standard statements

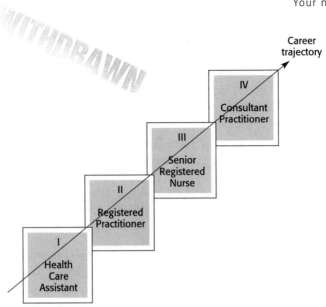

Figure 12.6 A career trajectory

related to care expectancy. Staff often did not know about them (other than the Patient's Charter), had not seen them or thought that they were in the back of a filing cupboard somewhere. Obviously a considerable amount of work is required in this area.

Strengthening leadership

The government recognises that nurses, midwives and health visitors need to develop leadership skills. In order to achieve this there will need to be a stronger focus on clinical leadership. While it is recognised that not all nurses, midwives and health visitors wish to become leaders, those aspiring to leadership need to be identified, supported and developed. Ultimately plans will be published to show how professionals will have access to wider programmes designed to strengthen leadership.

Modernising professional self-regulation

There is to be more open and streamlined regulatory framework with the possible regulation of support workers (discussed later in this chapter).

Working in new ways

Extending the roles of professionals to make better use of skills by modernising the roles of health visitors and school nurses, introducing more nurse-led primary care services and midwives taking on wider responsibilities are all aspects of working in new ways. Again this will require a considerable amount of work if it is to be achieved.

Overall this work will serve to move the various professions into the twenty-first century as it is enacted with the next document to be examined, *Fitness for Practice* (UKCC 1999).

Fitness for Practice (1999)

During March 1998 the UKCC agreed to the establishment of the Commission for Education. Sir Leonard Peach chaired the commission and so the report is often referred to as 'The Peach Report'. The work of the Commission was completed in August 1999 and its findings (Table 12.6) were presented to the board in September 1999. The purpose of the Commission was to prepare the way forward for pre-registration nursing and midwifery education that enables fitness for practise based on health care need. The commission members were conscious of the diversity of the present arrangements and the significance of the role played by the independent sector; similarly, student opportunities within a multiplicity of care environments were examined. The number of patients and clients treated, the range of health care needs, greater public expectations and new ways of providing care and delivering services all require flexibility and diversity. The commission states in paragraph 13: 'we do not believe there is merit in adopting a common approach to defining outcomes for pre-registration education pro-

Table 12.6 Abridged recommendations from 'Fitness for Practice'

1. Careers services should offer a breadth of advice, encouraging access for all.
2. Recruitment and selection should be a joint responsibility between health care providers and higher education institutes.
3. The good practices of organisations cooperating in providing entry through access programmes to pre-registration preparation should be extended.
4. The use of AP(E)L should be introduced within the CFP.
5. The CFP should be reduced to one year and should enable the achievement of a common level of competence. It should be taught in the context of, and enable integration with, the branch programmes and should introduce clinical skills and practice placements early in the programme.
6. Students who leave having successfully completed at least one year of the CFP should be able to benefit by mapping their academic and practice credit against other credit frameworks.
7. More flexibility should be introduced concerning the time of branch programme selection.
8. There should be an expansion of graduates' preparation.
9. A common definition of attrition and a required minimum data set should be agreed.
10. The standards required for registration should be constructed in terms of outcome competencies, should make the practice component transparent and should specify consistent clinical supervision.
11. The benchmarking of subject-specific standards should address outcomes that are core and specific to nursing and to midwifery, are transferable, and are consistent with the Quality Assurance Agency's threshold for degrees and diplomas.

Table 12.6 (continued)

12. Consideration should be given as to whether pre-registration midwifery education should move to a competency-based approach.

13. Students, assessors and mentors should know what is expected of them through specified outcomes and competencies which form part of a formal learning contract, give direction to clinical placements and are jointly negotiated between the health care providers and HEIs.

14. The use of a portfolio of practice experience should demonstrate a student's fitness to practise and evidence of rational decision making and clinical judgement.

15. The portfolio should be assessed through rigorous practice assessment tools.

16. The sequencing and balance between theory and practice should promote integration of knowledge, attitudes and skills.

17. The current programme model of four branches of nursing should be reviewed in the light of changing health care needs.

18. Practice placements should achieve agreed outcomes which benefit student learning and provide experience of the full 24-hour-per-day and seven-day-per-week nature of health care.

19. Interpersonal and practice skills should be fostered by the use of experiential and problem-based learning, increased use of simulation laboratories and access to information technology, particularly in clinical practice.

20. There should be a period of supervised clinical practice of at least three months' duration towards the end of the pre-registration programme.

21. All newly qualified registrants should receive a properly supported period of induction and preceptorship when they begin in their employment.

22. Programme changes should be systematically evaluated in respect of achieving fitness for practice.

23. Health care providers and HEIs should continue to develop partnerships to support students, curriculum development, implementation and evaluation, joint awareness and the development of service and education issues, and delivery and monitoring of learning practices.

24. An accountable individual should be appointed by education purchasers to liaise with health care providers and HEIs to support the provision of sufficient suitable placements, staff and students during placements, the development of standards and specified outcomes for placements, and the delivery and effective monitoring of the contract.

25. Health care providers and HEIs should work together to develop diverse teams of clinical and academic staff offering expertise in clinical practice, management, assessment, mentoring and research.

26. Health care providers and HEIs should support time in education and practice for clinical and education staff respectively to enable competence and confidence.

27. Practice arrangements should be made through appropriate channels.

28. Health care providers and HEIs should formalise the preparation, support and feedback to mentors and preceptors.

29. Funding to support learning in practice should take account of the cost of mentoring, assessment by clerical staff, and lecturers having regular contact with practice.

30. To improve workforce planning for nursing, NHS requirements should increasingly be informed by comprehensive information from the private and independent sector.

31. The government departments concerned with health, social care and social services, education and employment should work collaboratively to ensure that the preparation of health and social care assistants is based upon common standards of practice values.

Table 12.6 (continued)
32. The health care professions should be actively encouraged to learn with and from one another.
33. Consideration should be given to the most appropriate method of funding students of nursing and midwifery in future.

grammes to ensure that all newly qualified nurses and midwives are fit for practice'. It was therefore felt that both pre-and post-registration programmes should foster a climate of lifelong learning and continuing professional development (CPD).

It can be seen from the recommendations (Table 12.5) that some of the proposals can be implemented immediately whereas others will require further work. It is the belief of the Commission that, once the recommendations are implemented, programmes will prepare practitioners who are able to adapt to meet future health care needs. These recommendations should be implemented over the next few years; however, it may be longer before their impact is felt because the pre-registration programme is of three years' duration.

Post Registration Education and Practice

Post Registration Education and Practice (PREP) has been formulated by the United Kingdom Central Council for Nursing, Midwifery and Health Visiting (UKCC): it defines what nurses must do in order to maintain an effective registration on the different parts of the UKCC professional register.

Since April 1998 all registered nurses, midwives and health visitors need to demonstrate that they have met the UKCC's PREP requirements for study activity when they renew their registration. The purpose of PREP is to develop standards for a framework of post-registration education and practice which would contribute to the maintenance and development of professional knowledge and competence (UKCC 1997). The standards are:

- maintaining registration with the UKCC
- specialist practice

in order to improve standards of patient and client care both directly and indirectly. This will then demonstrate that members of the professions will not only have reached the required standard of initial registration but they will also have maintained and developed professional knowledge through additional learning activities, for the benefit of patient and client care.

Together with this, for those experiencing a break in practice of more than five years there will be a statutory 'return to practice' programme.

There are four key elements to maintaining registration:

1. Completing a 'notification of practice' form at the point of initial registration and every three years thereafter or when your area of professional practice changes to one where you will use a different registrable qualification.
2. A minimum of five days or equivalent of study activity every three years.
3. Maintaining a personal professional profile containing details of your professional development.
4. A 'return to practice' programme if you have not practised for a minimum of 750 hours or 100 working days in the five-year period leading up to the renewal of your registration.

Together with this there are five categories of study, which lend themselves to a number of professional development activities:

1. *Reducing risk*: This relates to clinical factors, setting standards and empowering patients. A practice nurse, for instance, might want to organise a path of study leading to the setting up of a smoking cessation clinic.
2. *Care enhancement*: Once again, this focuses on developments in clinical practice. Attending a workshop or conducting a literature review related to your clinical practice would be relevant here.
3. *Patient, family, clients and colleague support*: Clinical supervision and leadership counselling are just a few of the skills that come to the fore.
4. *Practice development*: This might include visiting a unit of interest that may affect the delivery of care within your practice area or it could mean studying articles related to the delivery of care in your area in order to enhance practice.
5. *Education development*: Devising personal programmes of study are again relevant.

Attending conferences or study days are not the only ways of learning; it is the evidence you present within your personal professional profile that is important. It is through this method of keeping a record that assessment will take place. It is worth noting, at this point, that the five days' study (i.e. thirty-eight hours, not five study days) is the *minimum* required in assisting you towards re-registration. No one has suggested that the five days in three years will enable you to reach your full potential but it will go some way to ensuring that your patients or clients will receive good quality care.

Personal professional profile

Your personal professional profile is a reflection of you as a person and as a professional. The physical shape of this profile will be decided upon by you, but it is useful to consider keeping a ring binder as this is probably the most flexible way of retaining the information you wish to be considered when you demonstrate your updating. Similarly, you might wish to keep a secondary binder in which you retain all evidence collected from the previous three-year period. This means that what is in your profile is current and relevant to the present time.

What should you include in your professional portfolio?

Record factual information, for example personal biographical details, professional registrable qualifications, other academic qualifications, posts held throughout your career and other activities that you may feel are relevant, e.g. PTA secretary or member. Indeed, these are the items that you might normally include within your curriculum vitae (CV). Together with this there should be some indication that you have appraised your professional performance through reflection (Chapter 4) and by identification of your strengths and weaknesses (Chapter 1); your achievements; also the clinical, teaching or management areas that you would wish to develop. You would also include evidence of each learning experience as you undertake it, the length of time it took to achieve your goal, and copies of goal and action plans (Chapter 1); reflection related to the effect that this episode of learning would have on patient care; and a record of the total actual hours you have utilised over the three-year registration period. It is worth remembering that your personal professional profile is your own property and your manager does not have the right to demand to see its contents; however, a verifier appointed by the UKCC has the right to examine all evidence of updating.

Every time you re-register you will be required to make a formal declaration to the UKCC/Nursing and Midwifery Council confirming that you have met the statutory obligations for PREP. You may not necessarily be required to produce your profile on every occasion, but the UKCC/Nursing and Midwifery Council retains the right to select a percentage of all profiles over the year.

Skills for the future

Can you think what skills for the future might be?

Problem solving, communication, professional judgement, collaboration and a sound knowledge base all spring to mind, in fact everything discussed in Chapters 1–4. Patient and client choice is important for future health care professionals.

What do patients and clients value in their health care professionals?

Milburn *et al.* (1995) conducted a small study looking at the type of care preferred. The study showed that patients valued: emotional support and understanding through certain actions; regular contact; listening to patients and allowing them to talk; treating patients as individuals, calling them by preferred names; working in a relaxed, informal, calm and friendly way with continuity of care. Patients also discussed the value of knowledgeable nurses, who were able to do things for patients who could not do 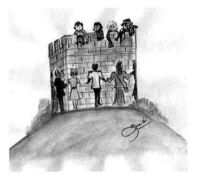 these things for themselves. Psychological care in terms of showing concern, understanding and knowledge of diseases and treatments was also seen as providing psychological safety. Explaining information given by the doctor was also emphasised.

Conclusion

This final chapter has set out to highlight and suggest the way forward by discussing further the elements required to maintain your registration and lead you on to a fulfilling career.

It is impossible, in a book of this nature, to cover all the elements of management in any great depth but it is hoped that this insight into management strategies and theories will kindle your enthusiasm for becoming an effective manager throughout your career.

Summary of key points

This final chapter has attempted to draw together some of the aspects of practising as a registered nurse, midwife or health visitor. Particularly it has examined the following areas:

- **Coping with the transition from student to qualified nurse, midwife or health visitor:** This factor is something you will have looked forward to since commencing your course. The potential problems were highlighted and suggestions for coping through effective preceptorship were made.

- **Career opportunities: the way forward, career paths, agency working:** Deciding the way forward is often difficult as during your training you will have been exposed to short experiences in a variety of settings. Also your needs may have changed in terms of availability to work so strategies were suggested where you will be able to adjust your working time to suit your personal needs. Together with this is the nature of the career path, whether it will be vertical or diverse.

- **Applying for your chosen role:** A potentially hazardous and worrying time. This sections dealt with coping and preparing for the rigours of the experience.

- **Practising in the New Millennium:** Identified the dilemmas highlighted within *Healthcare Futures 2010* in order to identify the way forward for health care provision.

- ***Making a Difference***: Nursing in the 'new' NHS described the government proposals to maximise the quality of the delivery of care in the future.

- ***Fitness for Practice***: Described the current document relating to nurse, mid-wife and health visitor preparation.

- **Post Registration Education and Practice:** Examined the need to maintain and develop professional knowledge throughout your career in order to con-tinue to practice.

- **Personal professional profile:** This is a mandatory element of notification of intention to practice. It is factual evidence of updating in line with PREP and it is a collection of your personal reflections on your own practice in order to enhance quality and standards of care.

- **Skills for the future:** Linked back to the initial chapters in the book highlight-ing the need for effective communication, professional judgement and a host of other skills in order to practise effectively in the future.

References

Buckenham M A (1988) Student nurse perception of the Staff Nurse role, *Journal of Advanced Nursing*, **13** 662–70

Department of Health (1994) *The Challenges for Nursing and Midwifery in the 21st Century* (The Heathrow Debate), HMSO

Department of Health (1999) *Making a Difference: Strengthening the Nursing, Midwifery and Health Visitor Contribution to Health and Healthcare*, HMSO

ENB (1993) *Guidelines for Educational Audit*, ENB

Hancock C (2000) Foreword, *Directions 2000*, Royal College of Nursing

Hanks P (ed.) (1983) *Collins English Dictionary*, Collins

Humphries A (1987) The transition from student to Staff Nurse, unpublished B.Sc. thesis, Leicester University, cited in Lathlean and Corner J (ed.) (1991) *Becoming a Staff Nurse: A Guide to the Role of the Newly Registered Nurse*, Prentice Hall

Hydes-Greenwood J, Sargent R (2001) All Together Now, *Nursing Management* **8** (2) 6-7

Kramer M (1974) *Reality Shock: Why Nurses Leave Nursing*, C V Mosby

Marquis B L and Huston C J (2000) *Leadership Skills and Management Fuctions in Nursing: Theory and Applications* (3rd edn) Lippincott

Milburn M, Baker M J, Gardner P, Hornsby R, Rogers L (1995) Nursing care that patients value, *British Journal of Nursing*, **4** (18), 1094 – 98

Moores (1999) in Department of Health, *Making a Difference: Strengthening the Nursing, Midwifery and Health Visitor Contribution to Health and Healthcare*, The Stationery Office

UKCC (1999) *Fitness for Practice* (Chair: Sir Leonard Peach) UKCC

Welsh Institute for Health and Social Care (1998) *Healthcare Futures 2010*, University of Glamorgan

Further reading

Bates T and Bloch S (1995) *Employability*, Kogan Page

Department of Health (1995) *Career Pathways: Nursing, Midwifery and Health Visiting*, HMSO

Department of Health (1995) *Creative Career Paths in the NHS, Report No. 4: Senior Nurses*, HMSO

Department of Health (1998) *A First Class Service: Quality in the New NHS*, The Stationery Office

Department of Health (1999) *Agenda for Change: Modernising the NHS Pay System*, The Stationery Office

Department of Health (1999) *Continuing Professional Development: Quality in the New NHS*, The Stationery Office

Department of Health and Social Security (1992) *Withdrawal of Guidance on Extended Role of the Nurse*, EL(92) 38 DHSS

English National Board for Nursing, Midwifery and Health Visiting (1996) *Return to Practice: Guidelines for Programmes Leading to the Renewal of Registration and Re-entry to Registered Practice*, ENB

English National Board for Nursing, Midwifery and Health Visiting (1997) *Post Registration Studies Programmes*, Circular 1997/01/RVL, ENB

Hart C (1994) *Behind the Mask: Nurses, Their Unions and Nursing Policy*, Baillière Tindall

Hopson B and Scally M (1991) *Build Your Own Rainbow*, Mercury Books

Hyde J and Wright A (1997) Self-development, *Nursing Management*, **4** (3), 10–11

Lathlean J and Corner J (eds) (1991) *Becoming a Staff Nurse: A Guide to the Role of the Newly Registered Nurse*, Prentice Hall

NHSE (1994) Networking: *A Guide for Nurses, Midwives and Health Visitors and Professionals Allied to Medicine*, Department of Health.

Puetz B (1994) Networking, *Public Health Nursing*, **1** (3), 174–7

Royal College of Nursing: Nurses in Leadership Project (1995) *A Guide to Planning Your Career*, RCN

Royal College of Nursing: Nurses in Leadership Project (1997) *Continuing Professional Development*, RCN Update, RCN

Royal College of Nursing (1998) *Guidance for Nurses on Clinical Governance*, RCN

Umiker W (1989) Networking: a vital activity for health care professionals, *Health Care Supervisor*, **7** (3), 65–9

UKCC (1992) *The Scope of Professional Practice*, UKCC

UKCC (1993) *The Midwives' Rules*, UKCC

UKCC (1994) *The Future of Professional Practice: The Council's Standards for Education and Practice following Registration*, UKCC

UKCC (1996) *Guidelines for Professional Practice*, UKCC

UKCC (1996) *Registrar's Letter 17/1996*, UKCC

UKCC (1997) *PREP – Specialist Practice: Considering the Issues Relating to Embracing Nurse Practitioners and Clinical Nurse Specialists within the Specialist Practice Framework*, CC/97/46, UKCC

UKCC (1997) *PREP and You*, UKCC

UKCC (1998) *A Higher Level of Practice: Consultation Document*, UKCC

UKCC (1999) *Protecting the Public through Professional Standards*, UKCC

UKCC (2000) *Positional Statement on Clinical Supervision for Nurses and Health Visitors*, UKCC

Useful websites

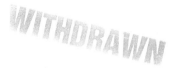

British Government	www.open.gov.uk
Department of Health	www.doh.gov.uk
English National Board	www.enb.org.uk
Health information on the Internet	www.wellcome.ac.uk/
Health Service Journal	www.hsj.co.uk/
Healthcare Informatics	www.healthcare-informatics.com/
Internet Journal of Advanced Nursing Practice	www.ispub.com/journals/ijanp.html
Journal Club on the Web	www.journalclub.org/allarticles.html
Management	www.dmsp.dauphine.fr/management
Medscape	www.medscape.com
Nursing Standard Online	www.nursing-standard.co.uk
On-Line Journal of Nursing Informatics	milkman.cac.psu.edu/~dxm12/OJNI.html
Practicing Nurse, the online journal for nurse practitioners	www.pracnurse.com
Qualitative Report	www.nova.edu/ssss/QR/index.html
RCN Support Services	international.office@rcn.org.uk
RCN Support Services	nurseline@rcn.org.uk
RCN Support Services	rcn.library@rcn.org.uk
RCN Support Services (RCN Wales Library)	angela.perrett@rcn.org.uk
RCN Support Services (RCN Scotland Library)	enid.forsyth@rcn.org.uk
Search engine	www.ask.co.uk
Search engine	www.copernic.com (this address is for a software company)
Sheffield University Nursing Site	www.//nmap.ac.uk
United Kingdom Central Council for Nursing, Midwifery and Health Visiting	www.ukcc.org.uk

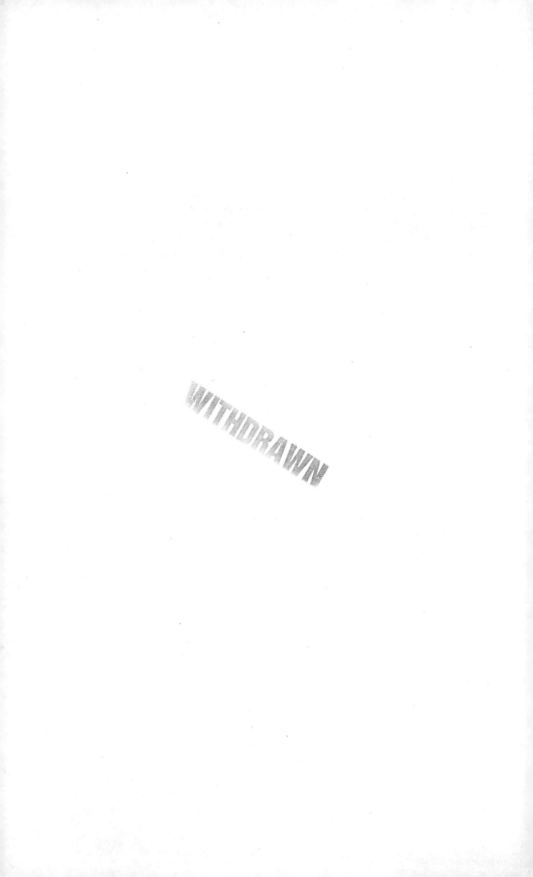

Index